PSYCHOANALYTIC CASE FORMULATION

Psychoanalytic Case Formulation

Nancy McWilliams, PhD

THE GUILFORD PRESS
New York   London

© 1999 Nancy McWilliams
Published by The Guilford Press
A Division of Guilford Publications, Inc.
72 Spring Street, New York, NY 10012
http://www.guilford.com

Printed in the United States of America

This book is printed on acid-free paper.

Last digit is print number: 9 8 7 6 5 4 3 2 1

Library of Congress Cataloging-in-Publication Data

McWilliams, Nancy.
    Psychoanalytic case formulation / Nancy McWilliams.
        p.   cm.
    Includes bibliographical references and index.
    ISBN 1-57230-462-6
        1. Psychiatry—Case formulation. 2. Personality assessment.
    3. Behavioral assessment. 4. Interviewing in psychiatry.
    5. Psychotherapist and patient. I. Title.
RC473.C37M38 1999
616.89—dc21   98-56044
                                                              CIP

For my husband,
Wilson Carey McWilliams

About the Author

Nancy McWilliams, PhD, teaches psychoanalytic theory and therapy at the Graduate School of Applied and Professional Psychology at Rutgers—The State University of New Jersey. A senior analyst with the Institute for Psychoanalysis and Psychotherapy of New Jersey and the National Psychological Association for Psychoanalysis, she has a private practice in psychodynamic therapy and supervision in Flemington, New Jersey. Her previous book, *Psychoanalytic Diagnosis: Understanding Personality Structure in the Clinical Process* (Guilford Press, 1994), has become a standard text in many training programs for psychotherapists, both in the United States and abroad. She has also authored articles and book chapters on personality, psychotherapy, psychodiagnosis, sexuality, feminism, and contemporary psychopathologies.

Preface

THE first time a supervisor asked me to venture a "dynamic formula-tion" of the case material I had just heard, I became instantly incompe-tent. I knew vaguely what I was being asked to do—namely, to suggest how the person's symptoms, mental status, personality type, personal history, and current circumstances all fit together and made sense—but I drew a blank as to where to begin. This was my introduction to the more interpretive, synthetic, artistic aspects of psychodiagnosis. Until I had been asked for that formulation, I had rarely in my training been encouraged to work inferentially, to open myself up to a creative pro-cess fueled by intuition, to feel my way into another human being's inti-mate life and formulate that person's suffering in a way that would express his or her unique categories of subjective experience rather than the preformatted, "objective" categories of received diagnostic wisdom. Like any well-socialized student, I had gotten good at memorizing fac-tual data, telling teachers what I thought they wanted to hear, and look-ing for the requisite number of "signs" that would either confirm or rule out a well-known diagnostic entity, but this assignment asked for something different and was initially very intimidating.

Most of us learn psychodynamic case formulation, as I eventually did, by identification with mentors who are good at it and who can demonstrate how better understanding produces better treatment. I am not entirely sure that this creative, affectively infused process can be captured in a book. But I was also uncertain initially whether psychoan-alytic character diagnosis could be effectively taught via the printed page, and I have repeatedly heard from students and practitioners that my writing on that topic has been helpful. So when my editor pointed out that in *Psychoanalytic Diagnosis* (McWilliams, 1994), despite my harping on the importance of sensitively assessing personality structure, I devoted only a footnote to how one arrives at such an assessment, I began thinking about how to convey in writing the ways in which experienced psychodynamic therapists think about patients.

They certainly do not think of them simply in terms of the criteria for "disorders" that are codified in the *Diagnostic and Statistical Manual of Mental Disorders* (DSM) of the American Psychiatric Association. To their credit, the authors of the DSM-IV have been explicit about the limitations of "disorder" taxonomies, especially from the point of view of the practicing clinician rather than that of the empirical researcher (American Psychiatric Association, 1994, p. xxv). To be a good therapist, one must have an emotional appreciation of individual persons as complex wholes—not just their weaknesses but their strengths, not just their pathology but their health, not just their misperceptions but their surprising, unaccountable sanity under the worst of conditions.

My previous book concerned the implications of personality structure for treatment. An appreciation of a client's character type is, however, only one of the factors that influences therapists in their decisions about how to work with someone. We want to know what stresses account for any person's coming to us at this particular time, how he or she has unconsciously understood those stresses, and what aspects of his or her unique background have created a vulnerability to this kind of stress. We also want to know how the person's age, gender, sexual orientation, race, ethnicity, nationality, educational background, medical history, prior therapy experience, socioeconomic position, occupation, living arrangements, responsibilities, and religious beliefs are connected with the situation about which we are being consulted. We ask about eating patterns, sleeping patterns, sexual life, substance use, recreations, interests, and personal convictions. We put all that together into a narrative that makes this human being and his or her psychopathology comprehensible to us, and we derive our recommendations and our way of relating to the client from that narrative (see Spence, 1982). Thus, in contrast to my previous book on diagnosis, this one concerns itself not just with those aspects of people's psychologies that comprise Axis II of the DSM but with data appropriate to Axes I, III, IV, V, and other areas.

This book is more about the process than the outcome of diagnosis. Even though there are numerous good sources on how to conduct an initial interview (e.g., MacKinnon & Michels, 1971; Othmer & Othmer, 1989), and several recent publications explicating different personality diagnoses or disorders (Akhtar, 1992; Millon, 1981; Kernberg, 1984; Josephs, 1992; Benjamin, 1993; Johnson, 1994), I am not aware of many primers on how therapists reflect on the deluge of information they obtain in a diagnostic interview—how they put it into not only a diagnostic formulation but also a general psychodynamic one. One notable exception is a guide by Paul Pruyser, who in 1979 not only described the process of psychodynamically influenced interviewing but also championed its importance with eloquence. Twenty years later, much has changed, both in psychoanalysis and in the culture at large. Currently, given pressures for quick, atheoretical diagnosis, it may be even more important than previously for those of us in the mental health business to remind ourselves of the complexities and subtleties involved in trying to understand people and their psychological problems.

I am hoping to reach the same audience I have addressed previously, namely, people committed to becoming therapists, whether their field is psychiatry, psychology, social work, counseling, education, pastoral work, nursing, psychoanalysis, relationship counseling, or the expressive therapies that involve the visual arts, music, and dance. Beyond the narrow goal of teaching practitioners how to develop and refine a dynamic formulation, I hope also to illustrate the value of the kinds of knowledge that constitute mainstream psychoanalytic expertise, and to provide support to my colleagues and students, so many of whom are suffering from the current, market-driven climate of cynicism about intensive and sustained mental health care. The public deserves therapists who maintain the integrity of psychological services and who resist letting economic pressures compromise either their commitment to a deep understanding of individuals or the compassion that naturally derives from that commitment.

Acknowledgments

THOSE who influenced my understanding of case formulation in direct, personal ways during my training include George Atwood, Bertram Cohen, Judith Felton Logue, Monica McGoldrick, Stanley Moldawsky, Daniel Ogilvie, Iradj Siassi, the late Silvan Tomkins, Duncan Walton, and my teachers at the National Psychological Association for Psychoanalysis, especially the remarkable Arthur Robbins. Psychoanalytic colleagues on whose expertise I continue to draw include Hilary Hays, Reid Meloy, Barbara Menzel, Gene Nebel, Arthur Raisman, Kit Riley, Jonathan Slavin, Sue Steinmetz, Diane Suffridge, and Bryant Welch. In addition, many seminal thinkers in the analytic community have been generous to me: The late Helen Block Lewis supported my earliest efforts to get my writing in print; Bertram Karon, Otto Kernberg, Stephen Mitchell, Fred Pine, Doris Silverman, and the late Lloyd Silverman all encouraged my work long before my professional reputation was established.

For continuing professional encouragement and promotion of my scholarship, I thank Stanley Messer, chair of the Clinical Psychology Program at the Graduate School of Applied and Professional Psychology (GSAPP) at Rutgers. Sandra Harris, Ruth Schulman, and my colleagues at Rutgers have made it a pleasure to work there. Jamie Walkup gave a draft of the first chapters of this book his typically thorough and thoughtful critique, much to its benefit. My students at GSAPP have contributed even more to my ongoing education than my fellow faculty members. I am also grateful to Michael Andronico and the members of my diversity self-study group—Clay Alderfer, Brenna Bry, Cary Cherniss, Lew Gantwerk, Bob Lewis, Hilton Miller, and Jesse Whitehead—for continuing to expand my consciousness into new areas of individual difference.

My understanding of individuality and its clinical implications is similarly nourished at the Institute for Psychoanalysis and Psychotherapy of New Jersey (IPPNJ). The hospitability of IPPNJ to open intellectual inquiry reflects the ecumenical tone set by my friend Albert Shire, its Director since 1984. Among my colleagues there, Karin Ahbel, Joseph Braun, Jean Ciardiello, Carol Goodheart, Tom Johnson, Linda Meyers, Marsha Morris, Lin Pillard, Jeffrey Pusar, Helen Raytek, Peter Richman, Jeffrey Rutstein, Helene Schwartzbach, Shawn Sobkowski, Nina Williams, and Sandra Yarock have been particularly important to my professional growth. Stanley Lependorf deserves special thanks for reading the finished manuscript under the pressure of a deadline and making useful suggestions for its improvement. My supervisees at IPPNJ and elsewhere, individually and in my private seminars, have consistently helped me to refine my thinking about case formulation.

Long before I was an analyst, I absorbed ways of conceptualizing individuality from Margaret Fardy and Dorothy Peavey, who educated me about, and promoted my respect for, personality types I have never seen discussed in official nosologies. Among my nontherapist friends, I am grateful to Cheryl Watkins and Richard and Brett Tormey for both cheering me on and keeping me humble, to Velvet Miller for her steadfast friendship over more than thirty-five years, to Nancy Schwartz for the warmth of her concern and the consolations of her wit, and to Fred Miller for his energy and his genius. As someone who finds meaning in play as well as work, and who needs the former to do the latter, I am indebted to Deborah Maher, George Sinkler, and the Copper Penny Players.

My most cherished mentor and supporter is my husband, Carey, to whom this book is dedicated. As a scholar of uncommon erudition, he appreciates the demands of the creative process and never complains when I am possessed by it. A feminist long before it was politically correct, he has always done at least half our homemaking and parenting, activities before which all other accomplishments pale. My daughters, Susan and Helen, have correspondingly expressed pride rather than resentment at my dedication to my work, making it easy for me to achieve without guilt. I also appreciate Theodore Greenbaum, Edith Sheppard, and especially the late Louis Berkowitz for what I have learned in their respective offices.

I have been fortunate to work with Guilford Publications. Sue Elkind, the prepublication reviewer for Guilford, improved this volume considerably. Kitty Moore, my editor, has now deftly guided me through all the stages of two books. She bears full responsibility for the existence of this one, having started to nag me about writing again when *Psychoanalytic Diagnosis* was still in press. When I protested that I had already said everything I had to say, she told me that had never stopped anyone else from writing a second book.

Finally, I thank my patients. It is so conventional for psychotherapists to say this that it is hard to do so in a way that sounds sincere, but I doubt that I am unusual among clinical authors in feeling a staggering debt to those who come to me for professional help. There are truths one can learn from a person who has been trying to bare his or her soul in increasing degrees of emotional nakedness over several years that no other kind of inquiry can access, and for these revelations I am grateful. Individual patients have kindly given their permission for the anecdotes about them in what follows. They have also confirmed that those vignettes are accurate depictions of their emotional experiences even though I have omitted or changed some data for their protection. Being a therapist is a fascinating, moving, and gratifying way to spend one's life, and I deeply appreciate those who have allowed me to do that job with them and who have in the process taught me most of what I know.

Contents

Introduction

THE ideas that comprise my thinking here were originally organized in response to an invitation from James Barron to contribute an essay to an anthology entitled *Making Diagnosis Meaningful: Enhancing Evaluation and Treatment of Psychological Disorders* (1998). In fact, this book is a much-expanded elaboration of that chapter, with a different audience in mind and a more complex collection of aims that I try to articulate in what follows. In his letter about the proposed book, Barron raised questions about tying the diagnostic process more meaningfully to the actuality of clinical work, about the complex relationships between diagnosis and prognosis, about the extent to which diagnosis informs treatment, about relating diagnosis to developmental processes, and about the tension between diagnoses that seek descriptive specificity yet obscure the complexity of patients and diagnoses that capture complexity but sacrifice specificity.

I have pondered such questions for years. As succeeding editions of the *Diagnostic and Statistical Manual of Mental Disorders* (DSM) of the American Psychiatric Association (1968, 1980, 1987, 1994) have become increasingly objective, descriptive, and putatively atheoretical, they have inevitably minimized the subjective and inferential aspects of diagnosis on which most clinicians actually depend. Operating more or less invisibly alongside the empirically derived categories of the DSM is another compendium of wisdom, passed down orally and in practice-oriented journals: clinical knowledge, complexly determined inferences, and consistent impressions made on the harnessed subjectivities of therapists. In any individual case, these data coexist somewhat uneasily with whatever formal diagnostic label the patient has been given. One aim I have here is to represent that invisible, shared set of procedures and reflections.

ON THE SUBJECTIVE/EMPATHIC TRADITION

From the perspective of an empirical scientist, human subjectivity is generally considered a detriment to accurate observation. From that of the clinician, subjectivity allows access to knowledge about human beings that one could never have of other subject matter (one presumes that physicists rarely "empathize" with particles). Many contemporary psychoanalytic writers (e.g., Kohut, 1977; Mitchell, 1993; Orange, Atwood, & Stolorow, 1997) essentially define psychoanalysis as the science of subjectivity, in which the analyst's empathy is the primary tool of investigation. Much of what I cover in this book reflects this subjective/empathic orientation. There is an important place for clinical observations made from this perspective, especially when they are scrupulously amassed and repeatedly compared with those of colleagues.

Several years ago, I agreed to be a research subject for a doctoral dissertation investigating differences in diagnostic preferences between psychoanalytic and cognitive-behavioral therapists. I consented to "diagnose in my usual way" certain material that would be presented to me on videotape. The tape purportedly showed a patient describing certain problems. I was to view it and then fill out a questionnaire. My immediate and persisting reaction to the video was that the woman describing her symptoms was not a patient; in her relationship to the camera, there was a complete absence of the usual emotional atmosphere one feels in the presence of a suffering person asking for help. I was quickly aware that I could therefore not "diagnose" her in the usual way I make clinical assessments—namely, by empathic immersion in the subjective experience of the person seeking a therapist's expertise and the disciplined exploration of what she provoked in my own subjectivity. The first item on the questionnaire was "What was your first reaction to the patient?" I responded, "That she was an actress, not a real patient." The subsequent questions, which assumed that the videotaped woman was in fact a patient, were impossible to answer.

I called in the student and explained to her my problem. I had been asked to diagnose in my "usual way," but my usual way required me to feel the presence of a person who was really asking for help. I said I was not trying to be difficult, but I could not fit my usual style of diagnosis into the demands of the experiment. The researcher confirmed that the videotaped woman was an actress but asked me to imagine anyway that she was a real patient. I said I could not do this: Diagnosis for me is not a strictly intellectual exercise, responsive only to described symptomatology. In exasperation, the experimenter decided to exclude me from her study, since I was not able to cooperate with her research on its own terms. The findings she later published simply omitted the assessment practices of therapists like me, who bring a more holistic, subjective, interactional sensibility to the task of understanding another human being.

Analogous omissions happen all the time with psychoanalytic data. Information is ignored because it is not "neat," objectively describable, full of discrete, observable behavioral units (cf. Messer, 1994). Therefore, it is no surprise that we have a lot of empirical data on cognitive-behavioral therapies and far less on psychoanalytic ones. Only a cognitively impaired individual could honestly conclude from this situation that cognitive-behavioral treatments work and that psychoanalytic therapies do not. We are missing data, but we are not in possession of data demonstrating that psychoanalytic treatments lack effectiveness. As George Stricker (1996) has remarked, we should not confuse the absence of evidence with the evidence of absence. What *can* be concluded is that we need to invest in the very expensive, complex, and creative research that psychoanalysis requires to establish its empirical status. Meanwhile, those of us who are already convinced of the efficacy of psychoanalytic work owe at least some account of our thinking.

In fairness to the critics of traditional therapy, there is ample evidence that psychoanalytic assumptions have often been mistaken (one thinks, for example, of some of Freud's more peculiar ideas about female sexuality), reflecting smug, culture-bound convictions that now look quaint at best, harmful at worst. Because of the limitations of lore, there will probably always be a healthy tension between the subjectively infused oral tradition and the objectively oriented syndromal one. Another source of tension is that practice often lurches ahead of research, for the simple reason that therapists, hearing from a colleague that a new technique can help patients, will try it before waiting for full empirical validation (the recent popularity of eye movement desensitization and reprocessing [Shapiro, 1989] or thought-field therapy [Callahan & Callahan, 1996; Gallo, 1998] come to mind here).

It is very difficult to do good research on conventional, long-term therapy, and few of us who feel the calling to be therapists also have the temperament of the dispassionate scientist (see Schneider, 1998, on the romantic tradition in psychology). We are not, however, indifferent to science. At least since the time of Spitz (1945), analytic practitioners have been deeply influenced in their practice and in their development of theory by controlled research, especially research in developmental psychology. Another aim of this book is to show how experienced analytic practitioners apply relevant research findings to the demands of formulating a case.

ON BEING A THERAPIST AND TEACHING PSYCHOTHERAPY AT THE TURN OF THE CENTURY

It is an irony of our times that at the point when psychotherapy has almost completely lost its stigma, at least in the middle classes, and at the point when a respectable literature on its effectiveness has accumulated (Luborsky, Singer, & Luborsky, 1975; Smith, Glass, & Miller, 1980; Lambert, Shapiro, & Bergin, 1986; VandenBos, 1986, 1996; Lipsey & Wilson, 1993; Lambert & Bergin, 1994; Messer & Warren, 1995; Roth & Fonagy, 1995; Seligman, 1995, 1996; Howard, Moras, Brill, Martinovich, & Lutz, 1996; Strupp, 1996), we are experiencing political and economic pressures that are demoralizing practitioners, discouraging clients from seeking help, punishing clinicians who are able to inspire patients' willingness to stay in treatment long enough to accomplish something enduring, and redefining as "therapy" a nonconfidential relationship that may be summarily stopped at any point (cf. Barron & Sands, 1996).

Becoming a good therapist is inherently arduous and time-consuming, but lately, the task has been complicated by anxieties among aspiring clinicians that they will not be able to practice the difficult art they have made so many sacrifices to master. As a teacher of therapists, I have seen evidence that these anxieties have been rising steadily in recent years. For example, in my introductory survey of psychoanalytic theory at Rutgers, I typically assign a paper asking students to analyze one of their dreams in classical Freudian fashion. Occasionally a kind of "class theme" emerges in the papers, often involving separation (students usually take this course in their first graduate semester) or self-esteem (not easy to maintain in graduate school). In a recent semester, almost half the analyzed dreams contained images of an intrusive, arbitrary, unempathic authority—hostile police officers, angry school principals, autocratic nuns, and the like. When I reported this pattern and asked class members how they understood its meaning, they associated immediately to their apprehensions about practice in a "managed care world" where some bureaucratic directive would suddenly override their clinical judgment.

If I had been writing this book fifteen years ago, it would not have the polemical edge it has now. We are in a period of painful crisis about health care in general and psychotherapy in particular. There has essentially been a corporate takeover of the health care delivery system, and like most health care professionals, I am highly skeptical about the applicability of corporate and commercial models to the helping professions. Although I find it hard to imagine that there will ever be a time when people will not want to talk to highly trained others about their problems, if perfunctory, insincere, and frustrating interventions are represented as psychotherapy, it will not be many years before significant numbers of people will think they have "tried therapy" and found it wanting. They are unlikely to think about trying it again.

These realities make it even more compelling for therapists to do their job conscientiously and effectively. If a client is restricted to a short-term therapy relationship, it is more important, not less, to operate from a sound diagnostic basis. If the job the patient wants done cannot be done under the conditions that a paying third party insists on, it is up to the therapist to be honest about that and to know how to convey to the client an understanding of that person's particular psychology and its therapeutic requirements—to impart a dynamic formulation in ordinary language (cf. Welch, 1998). Communications of this nature can themselves be understood or misunderstood based on how astute the therapist is about the patient's overall psychology.

It is a common contemporary belief, especially among managed care personnel, insurance company executives, and some academic psychologists, that psychotherapy, especially psychodynamic therapy, is wasteful and ineffective. The research that has been cited in self-serving ways by many third-party payers to justify the most minimal interventions in the name of treatment has consisted mostly of studies in which time-limited, identical interventions are delivered to carefully selected, randomly assigned patients with simple diagnoses, whose progress is evaluated strictly according to the fate of the specific symptom for which they came to treatment (see Parloff, 1982; Persons, 1991). As Seligman (1996) has pointed out, such procedures differ markedly from psychotherapy as it is actually practiced. Conventional therapy is typically open-ended, with the patient influencing time of termination; it is self-correcting, in that therapists readily change their approach when something is not working; it often reflects the client's active and discriminating selection of a therapist with whom he or she feels comfortable; it usually concerns multiple and interacting problems rather than isolated symptoms; and the therapist's and patient's criteria for outcome include not just symptom relief but improvement in general functioning.

Complicating matters, the rift between academic psychologists and dynamically oriented practitioners, for which both groups bear some responsibility, has affected the undergraduate and graduate teaching of psychology. Notwithstanding a few friendly university departments, the settings hospitable to psychoanalytic scholarship have been freestanding institutes and hospitals outside the academic mainstream. Because most academic psychologists have had scant exposure to analytically informed practice, theory, and scholarly research, their comments to students about the nature of analytic treatment are often wildly misinformed. It is not uncommon for individuals who earnestly want to learn how to help people to come to graduate programs in psychotherapy believing that psychoanalytic practice is represented by a withholding and authoritarian doctor, a worshiper of the mythic Freud, who says nothing for the first six months of treatment and then tells the patient she has penis envy. One impetus to my writing this book is my concern to bring the analytic tradition and contemporary analytic theories into classrooms where psychoanalytic ideas may not previously have been well understood or welcome.

Analytic psychotherapy is not a set of techniques that operate independently of those who practice it. Relatively untrained people with good instincts and a good heart can be effective therapists. Highly trained individuals who lack ordinary compassion can be disastrous ones. The art of the clinician is difficult to teach and especially difficult to convey to skeptics. Some people who disparage psychotherapy have no temperamental affinity for the sensibilities it involves. A relative of mine, a higher-up in an insurance company, tells me that unless they have a vivid personal or family experience with mental illness, executives in his line of work view therapy as a sentimentalized racket, ingeniously designed for the enrichment of its practitioners.

I have been struck over time with how many critics of psychotherapy have had a disappointing experience in treatment. They may have been diagnostically misunderstood or have gone to an incompetent clinician or have seen an adequate person who was simply a poor fit for them. If they were to get a bad haircut, these people would doubtless have fired their hairdresser rather than attack the profession of cosmetology. But so much is at stake in psychotherapy, so much is risked by the patient, that one can hardly react to its failure with a shrug and a change of plan. Grievances by those for whom therapy has been either useless or damaging are understandable. Nonetheless, it is exasperating to those of us who practice this difficult art to see our work distorted and devalued, for whatever reason. I hope this book exposes some of the difficulties, possibilities, and limitations of assessment and treatment in a realistic light.

Despite the fact that every therapist with a general practice treats only a small number of individuals suffering from each of the major kinds of psychopathology, by sharing knowledge, the therapeutic community has accumulated a vast amount of information about many conditions. Clinical experience generates many researchable questions; research will suffer if practitioners neglect to make explicit the premises from which they operate. I am trying in this book to convey ideas that the psychoanalytic community has developed over a century of conversations about patients, ideas that may be researchable in spite of not being fashionable in the current health care climate. I have also drawn on the existing research tradition in psychoanalysis, a tradition more substantial than many critics of psychoanalysis admit (see, e.g., Masling, 1983, 1986, 1990; Fisher & Greenberg, 1985; Barron, Eagle, & Wolitzky, 1992; Bornstein & Masling, 1998).

Although people of my generation have been chastised for having an attention span the length of a television commercial, I have seen no evidence that contemporary therapists are less eager than their predecessors to assimilate painstakingly accumulated clinical wisdom and clinically relevant research data. Yet given that market forces and academic politics are not always on the side of preserving complex and controversial truths, we can assume that therapists will continue to feel some isolation and will need to support one another in their shared knowledge and vision. I hope to contribute here to that supportive professional environment.

ORGANIZATION

The format of what follows is straightforward. After an introductory chapter on the relationship between case formulation and psychotherapy, there is a chapter orienting readers to the issues one faces in an intake session. The eight subsequent chapters address different aspects of psychoanalytic case formulation. Readers will be given rationales and procedures for assessing the patient's temperament and fixed attributes, developmental history, defensive operations, affective tendencies, identifications, relational patterns, methods of self-esteem regulation, and pathogenic beliefs. In all these areas, I try to show how knowledge of that feature of the person's psychology has implications for the therapist's approach to treatment. Those who wonder about my preferences in terminology and tone are referred to the comments about my choices in the Introduction of *Psychoanalytic Diagnosis* (McWilliams, 1994).

From Chapter Four on, I typically begin each chapter with some definitional comments and a historical review of psychoanalytic theory that bears on the concept under discussion. Usually, that means starting with Freud. I hope the reader understands that I do not do this out of some knee-jerk homage to The Father. Rather, I think it is hard for new therapists to understand the evolutions and transformations of classical psychoanalytic theory into the contemporary world of diverse analytic viewpoints without having some sense of Freud's original hypotheses. After these grounding comments, I usually talk about other analytic ideas on the topic and finally discuss how what I have covered applies to the therapist's choices about intervention. I have been liberal with case examples so that otherwise sterile concepts can come alive in the reader's imagination.

Because the message it tries to deliver concerns the intimate connection between good formulation and good treatment, this book is as much about therapy as it is about assessment. Like many committed therapists, I have a tendency to be opinionated about psychotherapy and to be deeply influenced by my particular clinical experience. I suspect that a passionate, perhaps even evangelical, sensibility is not unrelated to a therapeutic calling, and possibly to therapeutic success. This sensibility does not always correlate with evenhandedness. Other clinicians may disagree with many of the inferences I draw here. Therapists work effectively from many divergent perspectives, on the basis of different but ardently held convictions. If, irrespective of disagreements, my writing stimulates reflection about the connections between a careful dynamic formulation and the psychotherapy that follows from it, I will be satisfied that I have made a contribution to clinical practice.

CHAPTER ONE

The Relationship between Case Formulation and Psychotherapy

T HIS book represents an elaboration of my deeply held conviction that for therapy to be therapeutic, it is more important for the clinician to understand people than to master specific treatment techniques. I have nothing against technique, and in my own development as a psychotherapist, I have honed many useful technical skills. But I look with dismay on the current enthusiasm for generating "empirically validated treatments" ("EVTs") and teaching this collection of symptom-specific and manualized strategies as if it represents the essence of the psychotherapy process. The excitement over EVTs has created a growth industry in some sectors of the mental health economy—if you own the rights to a quick and empirically supported treatment for a problem that has attained a DSM label, you can probably retire tomorrow—but it threatens to do so at the cost of depriving beginning therapists of a vast and clinically invaluable literature on the treatment implications of any human being's individual psychology.

It seems to me self-evident that unless one understands someone's unique, personal subjectivity, one cannot infer the best treatment approach for that individual. What helps one person can damage another, even if the presenting problems of the two people seem comparable, and even if a particular strategy has reduced target symptoms in a statistically significant number of people in a well-defined pool of subjects with similar problems. As many clinically sophisticated observers have pointed out (e.g., Goldfried & Wolfe, 1996), the procedures and conditions that confer "empirical validation" on a technique are usually markedly different from the circumstances in which most practitioners work. And the current economic and political pressures to redefine psychotherapy as a set of short and symptom-targeted procedures are so patently incompatible with the intellectual and professional motivations of most practitioners as to be laughable.

But even putting aside the issue of whether contemporary trends in third- and fourth-party involvement are undermining good mental health care, there is an ongoing need for our training literature to explicate the bases on which most experienced therapists draw their treatment conclusions. I have felt for many years that psychotherapy is too frequently taught "backward," with a favored technique taught before a trainee fully appreciates the conditions that give rise to the need for that technique. Specifically, the student of therapy is told that a particular approach is the "best" or "true" way to reduce psychological suffering, with the explicit or implied codicil that patients who cannot conform to that way of working must receive "deviations" from the best technique or, worse, be rejected as untreatable. Psychoanalytic institutes have probably been more guilty of this than any other training organizations, with their common prejudice that psychoanalysis is the treatment of choice for anyone who is "analyzable," and that lesser candidates for treatment require rather unfortunate "parameters"— therapeutic "alloys" instead of Freud's "pure gold." But I have found comparable conceits in the trainers of family therapists, Gestalt therapists, rational–emotive therapists, humanistic therapists, and others. Often such teachers are relatively distant from the clinical trenches and have some personal interest in promulgating a particular approach. In a reasonable world, however, technique would be derived from an understanding of personality and psychopathology, not from the technical preferences of the practitioner (cf. Hammer, 1990).

In what follows, I talk almost exclusively about the implications of a good case formulation for psychoanalytically oriented treatment. I hope readers of other orientations will nonetheless be able to make the necessary translations into their own favored concepts and find the material applicable to their work. I have written within a psychoanalytic framework because I have always had a temperamental affinity for psychoanalytic theory, because analytic concepts constitute the professional language in which I have learned to speak, and because I have seen analytic therapy work. I do not think psychoanalytic treatment is the only way to help people, and in fact, I think a good psychodynamic case formulation can be an excellent basis for designing a cognitive-behavioral treatment or family systems therapy or other intervention.

Although I am a psychoanalyst, I find myself recommending family therapy, or relaxation exercises, or psychoeducation, or eye movement desensitization and reprocessing, or sex therapy, or a medication consult, or numerous other nonpsychodynamic interventions, depending on my understanding of a person's particular psychology. I send patients to behaviorally trained colleagues when I lack the skills to address a particular area of their suffering, and they send clients to me when they feel there is some personality issue operating that can only be addressed in long-term, intensive, analytic therapy. Most practicing clinicians I know do the same. What conscientious therapists have in common, despite their differences in favored theories and language, is their effort to understand each patient as fully as possible, so that they can make the most informed treatment recommendation. Assuming my readers share this attitude, let me begin by articulating some central psychoanalytic ideas relevant to case formulation.

BASIC PREMISES

In creating a psychodynamic case formulation, the interviewer's aim is usually to increase the probability that psychotherapy for a particular person will be helpful. There are, of course, other reasons to formulate a case, including a clinician's effort to give appropriate advice to staff dealing with a patient, or figuring out what to say to a patient's family, or making a good referral. But they are all related to working out the best intervention for the person whose psychology is being conceptualized. By understanding the idiosyncratic way an individual organizes knowledge, emotion, sensation, and behavior, a therapist has more choice about how to influence him or her in all these areas and to contribute to the improvements in life for which he or she has sought professional help. When we construct a formulation that seems to make sense of the diverse pieces of information we get in an intake interview, we do so with a view to exerting therapeutic influence on the patient's subjective world.

Because the whole point of a dynamic formulation is the development of interventions that will achieve certain therapeutic goals, it may be helpful for me to say a few things about the goals of psychotherapy as they are understood by most psychoanalytic practitioners. The fact that several of these goals are attainable only in traditional, long-term therapy should not deter clinicians with more circumscribed treatment possibilities from making careful case formulations; in fact, the shorter the time and the more compromised the circumstances in which one can do therapeutic work, the more critically important are the therapist's working hypotheses. I am emphasizing traditional goals for three reasons: (1) to orient those who are still able to do standard, open-ended psychoanalytic therapy; (2) to encourage those in less favorable situations to distill from these objectives what is possible and applicable in their settings, and (3) to give voice to a set of deeply cherished values that contemporary economic and political pressures have been undermining.

Despite the fact that psychodynamic therapists try not to moralize or to impose their personal views on patients, and despite the historical concern of analysts to avoid being enforcers of the conventions of particular cultures or subcultures, psychoanalytic therapy is not, and has never pretended to be, free of either basic assumptions or organizing values. When we talk about improvement in therapy (under which rubric I include both weekly, face-to-face treatment and more intensive forms such as classical psychoanalysis), we refer implicitly to a range of goals that go beyond relief of the specific problem for which a person has sought help. Some clients share the treater's broader vision of health and growth implicitly at the outset of treatment, and others come to it out of identification with the therapist during the course of their therapeutic work.

This vision of the objectives of therapy includes the disappearance or mitigation of symptoms of psychopathology, the development of insight, an increase in one's sense of agency, the securing or solidifying of a sense of identity, an increase in realistically based self-esteem, an improvement in the ability to recognize and handle feelings, the enhancement of ego strength and self-cohesion, an expansion of the capacity to love, to work, and to depend appropriately on others, and an increase in the one's experience of pleasure and serenity. In addition, there is empirical as well as anecdotal evidence that when these changes occur, other specific improvements happen as well, including better physical health and greater resistance to stress (Gabbard, Lazar, Hornberger, & Spiegel, 1997). A comment on each area follows.

GOALS OF TRADITIONAL
PSYCHOANALYTIC THERAPY

Symptom Relief

It probably goes without saying that the primary objective of psychotherapy is relief of the problem(s) for which the client originally requested treatment. It is my impression that symptom relief for most conditions occurs about as fast in dynamically oriented therapy as it does in other kinds of treatment. A patient's "presenting problem" or "chief complaint," which has typically become unbearable at the time he or she decides to give up commonsense self-treatment and consult a professional, often ameliorates or diminishes in severity once a therapeutic relationship is secure. Given the opportunity, people tend to stay longer in analytic treatment not because they are not getting help but because they are. Analytically oriented therapy tends to go on longer than therapy conducted in accordance with other theoretical orientations, because both client and therapist are pursuing goals of general mental health that go beyond the swift removal of a particular disturbance.

It is also rare that someone comes to a therapist with a single, delimited difficulty. The young woman with "simple" anorexia turns out to be enmeshed in a perfectionistic family in which her eating disorder is only one expression of her entrapment; the man who comes for short-term couple therapy to "improve his communication" with his wife turns out to have a secret lover who is rearing his unacknowledged child; the little boy referred for "acting up" with authorities has a private habit of torturing small animals. People rarely put their ostensible presenting problems in a detailed, confessional package when they come to a stranger; they prefer to feel out the therapy relationship before prying open their personal Pandora's box. In fact, many patients keep important secrets from their therapists for years, until they have built up enough trust to tolerate the anxiety that goes with revealing any area of deep shame, or until they have been helped enough in other areas to have a basis for hope that they could change in the area of the secret. Studies that limit subjects to those with a circumscribed, admitted complaint (as most studies of psychotherapy efficacy must do in order to zero in on a particular phenomenon) can shed only the weakest light on symptom relief as it actually happens in the field.

Finally, people typically come to analytic therapy because they want to get at the attitudes and feelings that underlie their vulnerabilities to particular symptoms. Sometimes they know this at the outset of treatment, and sometimes it is clearer to them in retrospect. One can often get someone to stop behaving in a self-destructive way, but it takes considerable time and work to get that person to a place where there is no longer a vulnerability or temptation to do so. People come to analytic therapy not just to get *control* over a troublesome tendency but to outgrow or master the strivings that are causing such a battle over control. The man who is compulsively unfaithful to his partner wants not just to stop having affairs but to be relieved of his constant preoccupation with fantasies about them. The woman with an eating disorder wants not just to stop vomiting but to get to the point where food is merely food to her, not a repository of desperate temptation and wretched self-loathing. A man or woman who was sexually abused in childhood wants to change internally, subjectively, from feeling like a sexual abuse victim who happens to be a person to a person who happens to have been a sexual abuse victim (Frawley-O'Dea, 1996).

Insight

Early in the psychoanalytic movement, there was an idealization of understanding as the primary route to emotional health. Freud's idea that the key to healing was to make conscious what had been unconscious derived both from his experiences of patients' symptomatic improvements when they were able to remember and feel things they had consigned to the unthinkable and from a general scientific positivism that assumed that to understand something was to master it. The equation of truth with freedom, an association at least as old as the oracle at Delphi (whose motto was "Know thyself") still pervades most psychoanalytic thinking.

Although contemporary analysts consider understanding, especially the affectively charged "Aha!" kind of understanding that has usually been termed "emotional insight," to be of immense therapeutic significance, they also credit numerous "nonspecific" factors (e.g., the therapist's quiet modeling of realistic and self-respectful attitudes, the client's experience and internalization of the therapist's stance of acceptance, the fact that the therapist survives the patient's seemingly toxic states of pain and rage) with just as much power. In fact, over the past couple of decades, almost all psychoanalytic writing about what is curative in therapy stresses relationship aspects of the treatment experience over traditional notions of insight (e.g., Loewald, 1957; Meissner, 1991; Mitchell, 1993).

Even the meaning of "insight" has shifted over the years from a somewhat static concept to a process embedded in relationship. In the "modern" age of psychoanalytic evolution, the term implied the attainment in therapy, via help from a dispassionate, objective practitioner, of an accurate understanding of one's personal history and a realistic appreciation of one's motives and circumstances (e.g., Fenichel, 1945). In these postmodern times, the term implies that patient and therapist have created together, from their combined subjectivities and the quality of the relationship that evolves between them, a narrative that makes sense of the client's background and predicament—a narrative truth rather than a historical one (Levenson, 1972; Spence, 1982; Atwood & Stolorow, 1984; Schafer, 1992; Gill, 1994). It is emblematic of current sensibilities that Donna Orange suggested for her recent book on psychoanalytic epistemology (Orange, 1995) the title "Making Sense Together."

Despite the dethronement of insight from its position as the sine qua non of psychological change, for analytic therapists, and for most clients, understanding remains a central goal. Both parties in the therapy relationship try to articulate the "unthought known" (Bollas, 1987). The analytic emphasis on understanding is partly attributable to the fact that the two participants in the work need something interesting to talk about while the nonspecific relational factors are doing their quiet healing. It may also reflect the fact that the kinds of people who seek to practice or undergo psychoanalytic therapies appreciate insight as a value in itself. Knowledge is thus pursued for its own sake in dynamic therapy, as well as for the sake of specific treatment goals.

Agency

In the preceding paragraphs, I mentioned the ancient conviction that knowing the truth sets people free. An internal sense of freedom is probably one of the most precious aspects of anyone's personal psychology. Most clients come to therapists because something is compromising their subjective sense of agency. They are being controlled by their depression or their anxiety or their dissociation or their obsession or compulsion or phobia or paranoia and have lost the sense of being master of their own ship. Sometimes they come because they have never felt in charge of their life, and they are beginning to imagine that such a state of mind would be possible if they were to get some help.

A respect for the client's sense of personal autonomy and an effort to increase that sense underlie many of the technical features of standard psychoanalytic therapy. For example, the sometimes exasperating tendency of analytic clinicians to throw questions back at their clients, asking, "Well, what do *you* think? How did *you* feel about that?" derives from this effort. So does the universal analytic practice of letting the patient pick the initial topic for each session. Or the general refusal to give advice if one's patient is at all capable of figuring out what is in his or her interest. The effort to respect, preserve, and increase the client's personal freedom takes precedence over most other considerations in analytic treatment (see Mitchell's [1997] characteristically thoughtful treatment of this issue).

When patients are asked retrospectively what they gained from a period of psychotherapy, their answers frequently feature an increase in their sense of agency: "I learned to trust my feelings and live my life with less guilt," or "I got better at setting limits on people who were taking advantage of my tendency to comply," or "I learned to say what I feel and let others know what I want," or "I resolved the ambivalence that had been paralyzing me," or "I overcame my addiction" are typical comments. In appreciation of the centrality of experiences such as this, analytic practitioners will generally impose their will on the client only as a last resort, usually when the person's life is at stake. Even in supportive therapy, in which suggestions are often made (see Pinsker, 1997), analytically oriented therapists make it clear that the patient is free to reject the practitioner's advice. Part of a good dynamic formulation thus involves an understanding of the ways in which a particular person's feeling of agency has been compromised.

Identity

In our current era, it is hard to believe that, just as the intellectual appreciation of childhood as a special condition did not emerge until the eighteenth century (Aries, 1962) and the notion of adolescence was articulated only at the end of the nineteenth century (Hall, 1904), the concept of personal identity as a formal theoretical construct did not exist until the middle of the twentieth century. Erik Erikson's (1950, 1968) work at that time offered to the sophisticated public a new perspective on a kind of problem that was beginning to be common in the postwar years. The concern that one had to "find oneself" and the suffering of "identity crises" were distinctive complaints of the 1950s and 1960s, as Eriksonian language about the struggle for self-definition captured the ear of a public looking to attach words to previously inchoate sensibilities.

Erikson, who had the advantage of having lived in an isolated Native American culture, was able to see how, by contrast, existence in a mobile, technologically sophisticated, mass society created unique psychological challenges. If I grow up in a stable, simple preliterate kinship group, as most human beings throughout history have done, the question of who I am is not problematic. I am the child of my parents, who are known to the whole community. If I am a boy, I will probably grow up to do what my father does; if I am a girl, I will become a woman like my mother. My role in my society will be clear, and though my options will be comparatively few, my psychological security will be reasonably assured. I will not have to worry about the meaning of my existence or whether I matter in the grand scheme of things. If, by contrast, I grow up in a huge country where I repeatedly deal with strangers, where I move from place to place, where I have no personal access to those with ultimate power and authority, where people I do not know give me conflicting messages through impersonal means of communication about how I should dress, what I should eat, how I should think, whom I should admire, and what I should do with my life, then the task of figuring out who I am and where I fit in all this confusion becomes critical (cf. Keniston, 1971).

I am exaggerating this contrast between simpler and more intimate cultures and our own complex and more anonymous one to make the point that developing a solid sense of identity has become an unavoidable aspect of contemporary psychological life. Even people growing up in the world's remaining tribal cultures are no longer shielded from technology and its mixed emotional blessings; the identity struggles of those in cutting-edge, cyberspace-savvy "developed" cultures are now shared by adolescents and young adults in the farthest-flung outposts of "civilization." Early in this century, if Freud's patients can be regarded as reflecting the spirit of their times, even urban people still seemed to know fairly well who they were. They came to Freud and other analytic pioneers to address conflicts between their conscious, relatively coherent sense of identity and their more subterranean wishes, drives, fears, and self-criticisms. Contemporary clients often come to therapy needing to formulate even their conscious sense of who they are.

The seminal works of Carl Rogers (e.g., 1951, 1961) and later of Heinz Kohut (e.g., 1971, 1977) spell out some technical therapeutic implications of the now widespread striving for a sense of identity: People need to feel understood, mirrored, accepted, validated in their subjective experiences. In the absence of dependable, predefined, lifelong roles offered by one's culture, one must derive a sense of who one is largely from an internal integrity and authenticity, a capacity to live by one's values and to be honest about one's feelings, attitudes, and motivations. In these times, experiencing one's identity solely by reference to connections outside the self is a dangerous practice, as people can attest whose jobs have been eliminated by the company that had defined them, or who have been recently divorced by the spouse who had given life meaning. In the absence of reasonably supportive contexts, people often need a therapist's help in their efforts to experience and verbalize who they are, what they believe, how they feel, and what they want. The effort to develop a strong and cohesive sense of self may be a person's primary preoccupation in therapy or it may exist more silently alongside other goals and concerns.

Self-Esteem

In even the most confident of people, self-esteem can be quite fragile, as anyone knows who has suddenly felt a good mood self-destruct in the wake of unexpected criticism. And even ordinary levels of reasonably robust self-esteem are much harder to promote than therapists would wish. Perhaps it is just as well that human beings are resistant to changing core beliefs, since we would all be much more subject to mind control techniques if we could readily be influenced to transform our deepest attitudes toward ourselves. Yet those of us who make our living trying to persuade self-hating people that there is nothing inherently wrong with them do wish we could do it faster. At minimum, we would like to ensure that we avoid doing any further damage to anyone whose self-esteem is already hanging by a thread.

One means by which a client's self-esteem increases in psychotherapy is the therapist's willingness to be seen as flawed. Both because it is the truth and because it models adequate self-regard in the context of imperfection, the psychoanalytic therapist conveys a conviction of having the capacity to help the patient despite acknowledged mistakes and limitations. In my view, the most important contribution of the self psychology movement to psychotherapy technique is its emphasis on the inevitability of the patient's disillusionment in the therapist and the importance of the therapist's admission of responsibility for empathic failure (Wolf, 1988). It is often a new experience for a client to see an authority maintain self-esteem while acknowledging imperfections and shortcomings. It raises the possibility that the client, too, can feel good about his or her less-than-perfect self.

Another way self-esteem becomes more solid and reliable in therapy concerns the patient's experience of unrelenting honesty, a commitment to the truth that insists that no part of one's experience be hidden from the self or the therapist. As the therapist accepts, often without even the need to comment, the client's most anxious and shame-drenched disclosures, the client starts reframing these areas of personal shortcoming as ordinary rather than terrible. Or as terrible but not the whole story of his or her personality. The support of people's realistically based self-esteem (as opposed to narcissistic inflation) has very lit-tle to do with saying nice things to them or "reinforcing" them for their observably stellar qualities. In fact, such remarks frequently backfire, as the patient silently muses, "My therapist is a very nice person who obvi-ously has no inkling of what I'm *really* like." Even in therapies that lack the advantage of adequate time to increase basic self-esteem, a dynamic formulation that captures the patient's particular self-esteem economy will permit the therapist to avoid unnecessarily wounding a person, as happens all too often.

Recognizing and Handling Feelings

When psychoanalytic theories first crossed the Atlantic and encoun-tered the American penchant for utopianism, numerous misconceptions filtered down to the public about the nature of psychological health, some of which are still around. One of the misconceptions that has faded in recent times but that enjoyed a great vogue in the middle of the twentieth century is the idea that the emotionally healthy person is "un-inhibited." The character of Auntie Mame (Dennis, 1955) gave lovingly sardonic literary form to a kind of enthusiasm prevalent among midcentury intellectuals to the effect that one should be liberated from sexual restraints and fully spontaneous in one's emotional expression. It was the stock in trade of many a midcentury seducer to imply that a woman who was not interested in sex with him was pathologically timid or "frigid." In the 1960s and 1970s, all kinds of therapeutic inno-vators, from the creators of Esalen to the advocates of primal scream-ing, idealized the spontaneous expression of emotion. In the climate of the era, thoughtful people who deliberated before they spoke were fre-quently branded as "up-tight" or "blocked." I bring these travesties up for the sake of contrasting them with the actual aims of psychoanalytic therapy, which has a lot to do with feelings but nothing to do with an ideal that they should always be freely and spontaneously expressed.

What one hopes will develop in psychotherapy is a set of sensibili-ties like those that Daniel Goleman (1995) has recently called "emo-tional intelligence," qualities that an older psychoanalytic tradition re-ferred to as "emotional maturity" (Saul, 1971); that is, practitioners want their patients to know what they are feeling, to understand why they are feeling that way, and to have the internal freedom to handle their emotions in ways that benefit themselves and others. In analytic psychotherapy, we invite clients to say whatever comes to mind, no matter how nasty, embarrassing, or apparently trivial it seems. We do this not because such an injunction is a prototype for how people ought to talk in social situations, but because therapy provides a unique setting in which everything that can be verbalized becomes the "material" of the work of understanding.

Analysts are not hedonists, nor do they subscribe to a doctrine of "letting it all hang out" verbally. They understand that if one is aware of one's sexual feelings, for example, one has a choice to handle them by masturbation, by sex with a willing partner, or by abstinence, none of which require disavowing the feelings themselves. The operative concept is choice. Similarly, if one is angry, the important issue from a psychoanalytic point of view is not to vent the anger in the moment but to notice the feeling and find some way to use its energy in the service of problem solving. (This frequently needs to be spelled out for patients, who worry that by putting them in touch with intense negative feelings, the therapist is creating a monster.)

Pennebaker's (1997) extensive research provides solid empirical support for the notion that openness to feelings is associated with physical and mental well-being. A surge of contemporary work in neuropsychiatry and psychophysiology (e.g., van der Kolk, 1994; LeDoux, 1995; Schore, 1997) has begun to give us a picture of what is happening in the brain when people are experiencing strong affects, and what are the temporary and permanent physical effects of being affectively overwhelmed or traumatized. Therapists have always distinguished between intellectual and emotional insight and have known from experience that to transform into verbal expression something that first manifested as an inchoate body sensation or a feeling of impending dread or a behavioral compulsion is the route to understanding and mastery of the problem. Now we have evidence that this process involves, among other things, the differences between emotional memory, stored in the amygdala, and declarative memory, stored in the prefrontal cortex. The process, and the concrete advantages, of getting "the words to say it" (Cardinal, 1983) is becoming physically describable, as Freud originally hoped and predicted (see Share, 1994).

Ego Strength and Self-Cohesion

A related area that many psychoanalysts emphasized during the middle of the twentieth century (e.g., Redlich, 1957; Jahoda, 1958) is the capacity of a person to cope with life's difficulties in a realistic, adaptive way. It has always been hard to understand how one child with many seeming advantages can deteriorate into complete helplessness every time something mildly stressful happens, while another with a much less ostensibly favorable history can find ways to cope effectively with conditions that would flatten most of us. One of the frequent background reasons for a person's seeking psychotherapy is his or her wish to change a tendency to "fall apart" when life gets difficult. The analytic term for the elusive capacity to cope despite adversity is ego strength.

The term derives, of course, from Freud's famous (1923) tripartite depiction of mental life. The *id* (literally, "it") was a designation he expropriated from Georg Groddeck for the striving, demanding, primitive, prerational, prelogical part of the self. The id is entirely unconscious, though its contents can be partially understood by attention to "derivatives" such as fantasies and dreams. The *superego* (the "above-myself") was his term for the moral overseer inside most of us—the conscience, the self-evaluator. It was understood to be partly conscious, as when one congratulates oneself for resisting temptation, and partly unconscious, as when one suffers in some way because of guilt that is out of awareness. Freud's use of the term *ego* (literally "I") was roughly synonymous with what most people mean by "self." But he also wrote as if the ego comprised a set of *functions* that operate partly consciously, as in ordinary problem solving, and partly unconsciously, as in people's use of automatic defense mechanisms.

This hypothetical construct, the ego, theoretically mediates between the demands of the id, the superego, and reality. In analytic parlance, ascribing to someone a strong ego means that he or she does not deny or distort harsh realities but finds ways of prevailing that take them into account. Bellak and Small (1965) described three overlapping aspects of ego strength: adaptation to reality, reality testing, and sense of reality. A person with good ego strength is by definition neither paralyzed by excessive or unreasonable guilt nor vulnerable to acting on passing impulses. Empirical researchers of a psychoanalytic bent have devised numerous ways of operationalizing and studying this concept and of evaluating ego strength via projective tests (see Bellak, 1954), but therapists tend to assess it in more global, impressionistic ways when interviewing a client.

With the rethinking of psychoanalytic metapsychology initiated by Kohut, the self psychologists, and the intersubjectivists, our language for talking about this phenomenon has been shifting. The terminology of Freud's structural theory, with its emphasis on the ego as a reified inner structure, is less resonant to many contemporary practitioners than language that refers to the self and its continuity and stability. The popular observation that some people "fall apart" under pressure or strain refers to a phenomenon that many current analysts call "lack of self-cohesion." In other words, some people react to stress with a sense of complete disorganization and fragmentation of their sense of who they are. Roger Brooke (1994) has described the signs of self-cohesion and its absence in deceptively simple and clinically indispensable terms.

A major nonspecific outcome of good psychotherapy is increased ego strength and self-cohesion. One wants a person to be able to confront difficult challenges without the internal experience of fragmentation or annihilation. One also hopes that after therapy, a person can tolerate temporary states of regression and destabilization in the service of growth, that he or she has developed the knack of "going to pieces without falling apart," in Epstein's (1998) felicitous phrase. One of my patients, over a fifteen-year but consistently productive therapy, moved from a tendency to withdraw into a delusional paranoid state whenever she was mildly stressed to a capacity to cope with life that made her a bastion of resourcefulness even when her husband became disabled, her income was threatened, and her daughter was diagnosed with a terminal illness. Although she still has some of the vulnerabilities she had when she started with me, she now handles them radically differently, with self-protecting, effective strategies that maximize her strengths. Recently, somewhat to my astonishment, one of her neighbors came to me seeking treatment, on the grounds that she admired her friend's resilience and had been surprised to learn about her treatment history.

Love, Work, and Mature Dependency

Freud (1933) stated that the ultimate goal of psychotherapy is the capacity to love and to work. Aside, however, from his implicit stress on the relationship between loving heterosexual attachment and acknowledging and giving up envy (in women, envy of male prestige and power, and in men, envy of female privileges to show passivity and dependency), Freud said rather little about love. Intriguingly, in a 1906 letter to Carl Jung (McGuire, 1974), he did comment that psychoanalysis was essentially a "cure through love," something he apparently regarded as self-evident. Later analysts, on the other hand, have discussed love at great length (e.g., Fromm, 1956; Bergmann, 1987; Benjamin, 1988; Person, 1988; Kernberg, 1995). This is hardly surprising, since it is to improve their love lives, whether heterosexual, homosexual, bisexual, or nonsexual, that people so often seek treatment.

When psychotherapy goes well, clients find that they feel more accepting not only of their complex internal lives and their "real" selves but also of the complexities and shortcomings of others. They see their friends, relatives, and acquaintances in the contexts of the others' situations and histories, and they take disappointments less personally. As they forgive themselves for things they now understand and can control, they forgive others for what they do not understand and cannot control. Having confided their darkest secrets to a therapist who has not been shocked, they become less afraid of intimacy, of being deeply known by another person. Having explored their hostile and aggressive side, they become less afraid that it will somehow damage those they care about. Having taken in their therapist's compassion toward them, they extend it to others.

The ability to work, to find one's creativity, to substitute problem solving for helpless lamentation also emerges from a good psychotherapy experience. Martha Stark's (1994) eloquent exposition of the mourning process in therapy, the movement from "relentless entitlement" to a mature acceptance of what cannot be changed (and a new capacity for addressing what can be) is only the most recent description of a familiar process of growth in treatment. As Stark explains, the initial phase of therapy involves the client's slow acceptance of the fact that his or her psychological problems reflect accidents of a complicated fate and endowment, not some personal defect or failure; the second phase involves the painful appreciation that even though this is true, no one but the client can be responsible for solving those problems.

Although people in the arts and in creative roles of any kind tend to worry that psychotherapy will rob them of their emotional energy (by resolving the neurotic issues that initially compelled their activity), they typically find that their artistry is less conflicted, more disciplined, and richer after treatment. In Gordon Allport's words (1961), their achievements have become functionally autonomous of the conflicts that spawned them, conflicts that, by the time they seek help, are only in their way. Chessick (1983), emphasizing the pleasures that emerge in both creation and recreation when therapy has been successful, suggested that the Freudian treatment goals of love and work should be amended to "love, work, and play."

In his earliest theories, Freud stressed the centrality of sexuality in human motivation. Later, impressed by the evidence of human destructiveness (especially during World War I), he acknowledged aggression as a primary drive of equal power. Temperamentally a dualist, he explained most human behavior in his later works on the basis of a tension between *eros,* the life instinct, and aggression or *thanatos,* the death instinct. In this paradigm, love is the benign and creative expression of the sexual drive, and work, the positive expression of the aggressive drive. Freud's successors in the object relations movement have added a critical third "instinct" (if anything so complicated can still be termed as such), namely, dependency (attachment).

Freud tended to talk about people as if they were self-contained, individual systems. But beginning theoretically with Fairbairn's (1952) challenge to classical Freudian theory, in which he argued that infants seek not drive satisfaction but relationship, and empirically with Bowlby's (1969, 1973) studies of attachment and separation in infants, analysts have become increasingly impressed with the ubiquity of human connection, of our embeddedness in an interpersonal system where our sexual and aggressive nature is only part of the story. A huge literature on attachment has appeared during the last generation, as researchers and clinicians are repeatedly confronted with the evidence of people's lifelong needs for objects and arenas for their various passions. A related emphasis among self psychologists concerns the permanence of people's need for "selfobjects," those who mirror and validate us.

All this relates to one other outcome of effective psychodynamic therapy, namely, the transformation of infantile dependency into mature adult dependency. Western myths about human independence notwithstanding, we all need each other in both emotional and practical ways throughout the lifespan. Psychotherapy does not take dependent people and make them independent; rather, it makes them capable of handling their natural dependency in their best interests. It confronts counterdependent people with their legitimate needs for others. The main differences between attachment in infancy and attachment in adulthood are that unlike adults, children cannot choose those on whom they depend, cannot ordinarily leave inadequate caretakers, and have insufficient power to influence their objects to change their behavior. Many adults come to therapy feeling like children trapped in destructive relationships and concluding that there is something dangerous about their need for others. Ideally, they figure out during treatment that it is not their basic needs that have been problematic but their handling of them.

Pleasure and Serenity

The final goals for a psychodynamic therapy that I want to discuss briefly are perhaps the most elusive to articulate. Despite the fact that most of us think we know what is meant by the term "happiness," we are often rather self-defeating in pursuing it. Part of the blame for this can be laid on myths that permeate a commercial, market-oriented culture like ours, in which we hear unrelenting messages about how better bodies and more lavish possessions will save us from despair. In an individualistic, competitive culture, the promise is ubiquitously made that we each will be happy if we only have what we want. In many non-Western cultures, by contrast, the prevailing wisdom concerns how to learn to want what one has.

Psychoanalytic thinking is a curious blend of these sensibilities: It is thoroughly Western, positivistic, individualistic, and (originally, at least) concerned with drive satisfaction and frustration. Yet from the very beginning, there has been an emphasis on deference to the "reality principle," to delay of gratification, to becoming "civilized" so that one hangs one's self-esteem on one's contribution to the larger community and can renounce immediate satisfactions in favor of more deeply nourishing, lasting kinds of pleasure. As Messer and Winokur (1980) concluded, the psychoanalytic worldview is tragic rather than comic (in the technical, not the popular sense of these terms). Analysts emphasize how deeply conflicted we are, how we have to give up our infantile wishes, how we have to compromise. With the general move toward more relational models of human psychology and psychoanalytic treatment, where attachment and separation are even more important concepts than drive and conflict, a focus on mourning has replaced an emphasis on striving.

A good dynamic formulation will illuminate the ways in which a person thinks happiness can be pursued and will consequently contain implications for intervention. People's pathogenic beliefs and individual ways of supporting their self-esteem are often radically at odds with their prospects for genuine pleasure and contentment. Grieving over what is not possible sets the stage for enjoying what is. Very often, in the later phases of psychotherapy, a client will comment that while he or she had known previously what it was like to feel "high" or "in a good mood," the overall peace of mind that evolved quietly during treatment was something he or she could not even have imagined. Just as orgasm is inconceivable to those without sexual experience, or the thrill of having a baby cannot be imagined until one becomes a parent, genuine serenity is probably inconceivable emotionally to the person who has settled for temporary bursts of elation.

CASE FORMULATION FOR THERAPEUTIC
RATHER THAN RESEARCH PURPOSES

With the preceding objectives in mind, it becomes clear that what a therapist is doing when he or she makes a dynamic formulation is a very different process from the symptom-matching exercise that comprises diagnosis in accordance with the DSM. As I have argued elsewhere (McWilliams, 1998), therapists and researchers bring very different sensibilities to the diagnostic process. For example, therapists become impressed in their work with how many communications occur through facial expression, body language, tone of voice, pregnant silences, seemingly innocent questions, lateness, patterns of payment, enactments, and other nonverbal nuances that require a disciplined subjectivity to decode. They learn to trust the clinical hunch. The efforts of the creators of the DSMs ever since DSM-III (1980) to rid diagnosis of subjectivity so that researchers can share objective measures of psychopathology have increased the reliability of diagnosis but have not contributed to its validity (Blatt & Levy, 1998; Vaillant & McCullough, 1998). Subjectivity is critical for discerning the *meaning* of a particular behavior.

The Personality Disorders section of the DSM-IV is acknowledged even by enthusiasts of that document to be problematic. A repeated complaint is that when a person meets the criteria for one of the official categories, he or she usually meets those for one or more of the others (Nathan, 1998). In other words, the delineation of behaviorally defined pathologies of character in the DSM has not succeeded in discriminating types of character pathology very well, much less in capturing the uniqueness of anyone's particular "disordered" personality. Nor should we expect a nosology like the DSM to be capable of doing so (see Clark, Watson, & Reynolds, 1995). The art of developing a dynamic formulation is, like other arts, not formulaic.

Researchers in the empirical, positivistic tradition use parsimony as a criterion of explanation, while practitioners are repeatedly impressed with multiple and overlapping causation, or what Waelder (1960) called "overdetermination" (see Wilson, 1995). In other words, in a research project, one tries to isolate variables so that a particular cause-and-effect process can be exposed, uncontaminated by other possible explanations. In understanding the meaning of a problematic behavior, in contrast, one typically finds many contributants, none of which alone would have created the symptom. Anything important enough to have become a major problem to a person is usually overdetermined, not caused by a discrete variable. For example, an obese patient of mine had to become aware of all of the following contributants to her weight problem before she could successfully diet and keep the pounds off: a probable constitutional inclination toward overweight and some hypoglycemic tendencies; a mother who was overconcerned with her eating habits (beginning with feeding her baby on a rigid schedule and later acting hurt if she failed to eat everything on her plate); a family pattern of using food to distract from anxiety and shame (the mother would bring out a cheesecake whenever someone was upset); an identification with a beloved obese grandmother; a childhood molestation in which she had been victimized but for which she had been blamed (leading her to want to demonstrate graphically in her appearance her lack of seductiveness); a pattern of sadness and loneliness that were assuaged by the ritual of coming home after school and comforting herself with snacks; the development of a defiant self-image as a person whose self-esteem inhered in intelligence rather than in physical vanity; and a witnessing of her father's wasting death from cancer, an experience that had created in her the unconscious conviction that losing weight was a precursor to and cause of death.

In analytic therapy, it is the unraveling of many different strands of causation that eventually permits patients to get mastery over patterns they seek to change. Therefore, when trying to come to an understanding of a complex human being and his or her complex difficulties, a therapist is silently pondering several related questions while drawing out and listening to the client. I have organized the rest of this book around those questions that I think are the most pertinent to a good dynamic formulation. They are not exclusive, but if the clinician knows something about each of them, he or she will know a great deal of importance for helping the client transform suffering into mastery. They include the following areas of the person's psychology: (1) temperament and fixed attributes, (2) maturational themes, (3) defensive patterns, (4) central affects, (5) identifications, (6) relational schemas, (7) self-esteem regulation, and (8) pathogenic beliefs.

In understanding the obese patient I have just described, it was thus important to discover with her (1) that she needed to develop particular strategies for counteracting her constitutional inclinations toward overeating and to change her meal pattern to accommodate to her hypoglycemia; (2) that she had learned in the earliest phase of development that she had better eat everything now, because food would be unavailable for the next four hours, and in later phases that not finishing her meals would injure her mother; (3) that she must replace eating with other means of handling anxiety; (4) that she could soothe herself when she was unhappy and lonely by taking a hot bath, calling a friend, or going shopping, and that, ultimately, by grieving over the many unfortunate aspects of her life, she could emerge from her chronic sadness; (5) that she believed she would magically have her grandmother's positive qualities if she had her obesity (and conversely, that she would avoid her mother's negative ones if she avoided being thin like her); (6) that she was still living in a posttraumatic mental state in which she saw others as potential molesters and blamers; (7) that the value system by which she had supported a fragile self-esteem as a teenager was now operating to deter her from enjoying and profiting from a normal degree of vanity; and (8) that whenever she lost a few pounds, she became unconsciously panicky that she would die like her father.

I should stress that it is only in retrospect that all these determinants and their therapeutic implications are so clear. Some of the features of this woman's psychology were among my original hypotheses, while others emerged during the therapy process, surprising both her and me. Usually, a therapist has a few interconnected ideas about the sources of a particular client's suffering and finds that while investigating in those areas, all kinds of other realms open up. A dynamic formulation is only the roughest kind of mapping of someone's individuality, but it is essential to have some kind of map before we invite a person into a terrain where both parties could otherwise get lost.

SUMMARY

Psychodynamic case formulation attempts an understanding of a person that will inform the direction and tone of treatment. It is a more inferential, subjective, and artistic process than diagnosis by matching observable behaviors to lists of symptoms. It assumes a concept of psychotherapy as involving not only symptom relief but also the development of insight, agency, identity, self-esteem, affect management, ego strength and self-cohesion, a capacity to love, work and play, and an overall sense of well-being. I have argued that an interviewer can generate a good tentative formulation of a person's personality and psychopathology if he or she attends to the following areas: temperament and fixed attributes, maturational themes, defensive patterns, central affects, identifications, relational schemas, self-esteem regulation, and pathogenic beliefs.

CHAPTER TWO

Orientation to Interviewing

Before I go into the specific areas I enumerated in Chapter One as essential for understanding individual applicants for psychotherapy services, let me sketch out the underlying values and associated mechanics of clinical interviewing as I have come to view them. There are several good books available on how to do an intake interview, but few of them are oriented toward a specifically psychoanalytic understanding of the person coming for help. Moreover, most of them are concerned with the accurate labeling of a person's problem but not with the connection between a label and the establishment of a therapeutic relationship. That connection is the main focus of this book.

Readers who want a basic introduction to the traditional psychoanalytic approach to case formulation would do well to read Messer and Wolitzky (1997) on the topic. Those who have not been trained in clinical interviewing may find some help in the appendix in my previous book (McWilliams, 1994), where there is an outline of the topics that most conscientious therapists inquire about when meeting with a prospective patient. This rather comprehensive inventory, however, is both under- and overinclusive. It lacks some items one would ask about if the client had certain symptoms, and at the same time, I doubt that I have ever interviewed anyone with whom I have probed every topic covered in that outline. The back-and-forth quality of an early session, in which the therapist not only asks questions but also defers to the patient's agenda for the meeting, militates against a slavish adherence to a format. I would not want to go to a practitioner who doggedly followed an outline rather than sitting back and listening to me describe my own understanding of my problems and their sources and ramifications.

When I read other therapists' writing, I am often exasperated that they do not give the details of what they actually do and say with clients. With a few notable exceptions, they speak in generalities and in theoretical rather than descriptive language. To spare others that kind of exasperation, I have taken pains in what follows to be very concrete. Later in this book, I will comment on numerous theoretical matters that have practical clinical implications, but in this chapter, I try simply to represent the process of clinical interviewing, including the issues that influence how therapists tend to structure this process.

MY OWN STYLE OF INITIAL INTERVIEWING

I have been asked many times since *Psychoanalytic Diagnosis* was published just how I go about getting the information from individual patients that permits the kind of characterological inferences I explored in that book. I have been hesitant to present my own process as an exemplar of standard clinical practice, because it seems to me that every therapist develops a style of interviewing that is appropriate to his or her personality, temperament, convictions, training, and professional situation. My own way of working with people is idiosyncratic, reflecting all these things, and may be a poor model for a different kind of person in a different situation. But in sympathy with readers' curiosity about how therapists actually work, and in view of the relative dearth of self-disclosing accounts of what treaters explicitly say to patients, I offer the following as a description of my usual pattern of initial interviewing. Most of my patients who read it will probably protest that I did not do it just that way with them, and they will be right, but it is nonetheless the framework that is in my head and that orients me.

The reader should keep in mind that my clinical situation is a private practice arrangement in a home office. When my schedule does not permit my taking on a new client, I tell callers as much. Then I ask if they want to see me anyway for an hour, so that I can get a sense of them and their needs, with the aim of making an informed referral. When I do have openings, those who come for an initial interview assume that they will be able to work with me unless during our meeting they feel the chemistry between us is not good. Thus, unlike some clinics in which there is an intake process separate from a psychotherapy referral, in my practice, the intake session is usually the beginning of the ongoing relationship between the patient and me. Most of the people who come to me are voluntary and self-referred, and although this group contains a fair number of individuals with borderline and psychotic psychologies, few of the prospective clients who appear at my door are frighteningly disorganized or dangerous, or in need of immediate hospitalization.

My first contact is typically over the telephone: The interested party calls and usually states his or her reasons for considering therapy. I listen for a few minutes, make some comments intended to show that I have assimilated the information the person has given me, attempt to establish a warm connection, and then try to schedule a time when we can get together. I give directions to my office and take the person's phone number in case some unforseen event occurs, necessitating that I reschedule. If the caller has a question about my fee or my training or my orientation, I answer it, though sometimes I subsequently try to find out why that issue is on the person's mind. If the first contact comes via a message on my voice mail, when I call back, I identify myself as "Nancy McWilliams" rather than "Dr. McWilliams," because someone other than the prospective client may answer the phone, and for all I know, the person interested in my services is keeping from family members the information that he or she has sought treatment. I figure that in such cases, "Who's Nancy McWilliams?" is an easier question for the secretive client to field than "Who's this doctor who's calling you?"

At the time of the appointment, I shake hands, show the person in, and invite him or her to sit wherever would be comfortable, explaining that I will sit at my desk because it is easier for me to take notes there. I ask, "So how can I help you?" Then I listen. As long as the prospective client is talking in a communicative way, I say very little. If I find myself with a shy or inhibited person who has trouble talking, I ask a lot of questions and help to fill in what may otherwise be painful silences. I assume that the more I can reduce the person's anxiety, the better. It is frightening to tell one's troubles to a stranger, and whatever I can do to make it less so, I do. I generally take copious notes, for purposes of both recording important information and giving myself a task that distracts me from my own anxiety about a new situation.

After about forty-five minutes, I ask how the person feels talking with me, and whether he or she anticipates feeling comfortable working with me. During the last few minutes of the meeting, I want to accomplish several things: (1) to show the person I have been listening and have a feel for his or her suffering; (2) to assess the person's reactions to whatever notions I have about how to make sense of the problems described; (3) to convey hope; (4) to make a contract about regular appointment times, length of meetings, payment, cancellation policy, insurance arrangements, and the diagnosis to be submitted if a third party is involved. Some practitioners have the main features of the contract written out on an information sheet that they give to each client.* I have not adopted this procedure yet, but for reasons of both clarity and liability, it is probably a good idea, especially if one's practice includes a number of borderline, psychotic, and otherwise disorganized people. Finally, I invite any concerns that the person wants to have addressed before plunging into the therapy proper, and except when such questions feel too intrusive, I answer them. Unless the patient has in the course of the hour gone into most of the background areas I would ordinarily investigate, I then tell him or her that during the next session I would like to take a complete history, so that I will have a context in which to understand his or her problems. My rationale for each of these practices follows.

Inviting the Client's Reaction to the Therapist

The question about how the prospective patient feels talking to me, in addition to its concrete objective of our deciding whether or not to work together, is intended to send the message that I will be interested in how he or she experiences our relationship. It opens the door to any underlying transference concerns that have not yet been obvious (e.g., "I'm feeling pretty comfortable, which is strange, because I thought it would be hard to talk to a female authority about this"). And it alerts the client to the collaborative nature of therapy; that is, it implicitly emphasizes that I am the person's employee, that I want to do a good job, that he or she has the right to evaluate me or fire me if things do not feel basically positive between us.

From my perspective, despite the transference needs of the patient and the narcissistic needs of the clinician, a therapy relationship—at least in a private practice setting where there is provider and patient autonomy—is essentially reciprocal. The patient takes care of me by paying my fee. I take care of the patient by trying to understand and help. Unlike friends, relatives, and others who may have tried to help the client so far, I expect no emotional support in return. Psychotherapeutic treatment is thus by no means a "paid friendship," despite what has been alleged by some critics of therapy (e.g., Schofield, 1986). In friendship, there is reciprocity in that both parties make personal disclosures, both take care of the other emotionally, and both get taken care of by

---

*See Appendix for an example of such a written contract.

the other. The reciprocity in psychotherapy is the exchange of financial support for emotional support and expertise, an arrangement with human equality but not structural equivalence.

Conveying Understanding

When people come to a therapist, they are usually afraid of being judged, misunderstood, or treated with a subtle professional contempt. They often regard their own symptoms with bewilderment and shame, seeing them as evidence of a vague craziness that makes no sense. One of the first things I try to convey is that their problems are not incomprehensible. The first session is no time for confident, elaborate interpretations, but it often helps the client greatly for the therapist to say something like, "I can see why, given what you say about your father, the situation with your boss was so difficult for you," or "I notice it's exactly ten years since your husband's death, so it's possible your depression is an anniversary reaction," or "These intrusive thoughts you've been having are a common aftereffect of trauma."

When I make statements such as these in an initial meeting, I do it tentatively, as if I am applying my expertise in an exploratory way and inviting the client to let me know if I am on the right track. The more disturbed a person is, the more critical is this aspect of the connection. Very often, significantly troubled people have been told nothing more than that they have a "chemical imbalance" or a "genetic defect," with no further information to the effect that whether or not this is true, there are reasons why they are suffering more at this particular time, and there is a potential for them to be significantly helped by talk therapy. They come to a psychotherapist feeling defective, and they are surprised to learn that there are ways of thinking about what they have been through that make their psychopathology comprehensible to another person. I recommend Harry Stack Sullivan's work (e.g., 1954) to anyone who needs to have a feel for the tone and orienting values of this kind of communication.

Assessing the Patient's Reactions to One's Tentative Formulations

How the person responds to my effort to communicate a preliminary understanding of the problems he or she has brought to me indicates a great deal about how the client will work in treatment. Some people are immediately compliant, others immediately oppositional; some feel criticized, while others feel that the therapist has demonstrated a deep empathy. Some individuals cannot absorb any interpretation because it feels to them as if the treater is humiliating them with the demonstration that he or she has superior knowledge. Others feel that if all the therapist is going to do is to make empathic, facilitative reflections, they might as well be talking to a stuffed animal.

Every person is different with respect to how much he or she can accept from a therapist. When I was a patient in analysis, it was important to me to figure out everything I could by myself. Such an attitude reflected my rather counterdependent personality. I needed the analyst's presence and the data of my transference reactions, but especially in the early phases of my treatment, I preferred the sense of discovery to the situation of confirming or disconfirming someone else's interpretation. (Eventually, I made a lot of progress understanding and changing my counterdependency and became more interested in what my analyst had to say, but this took a couple of years.) The silence and discipline of a very classical kind of analysis was thus ideal for me. I was surprised when I began to practice as an analyst, however, that most people wanted more input from me than I had wanted from my therapist. In fact, they felt quite forsaken when I encouraged them to struggle alone to come to their own understandings. In an initial session, one wants to get some sense of how interpretations will be received, so that one can adjust one's style of clinical interaction to the particular needs of the patient.

Conveying Hope

Individuals who confidently expect a therapist to help them are probably in a small minority. Most people come to treatment having tried all kinds of approaches to address their psychological difficulties, from denial to willpower to self-help books and herbal remedies, and nothing has worked. Therapy is typically a last resort, to which they come with significant demoralization and cynicism. And however much we venerate our profession, it would be self-deluded for practitioners to believe that the general public has a high opinion of mental health professionals. Psychotherapists are widely seen—not without some justification—as individuals with serious psychological troubles, who feel better reminding themselves that other people are crazy too. Most incoming patients consequently are deeply skeptical about what we can offer them. Still, once they meet an actual therapist and find him or her to be a seemingly sane, competent human being, they may be able to access some optimism.

Sometimes it is a relieving surprise to a new client for the therapist to say, simply, "I think I can help you." I usually find myself saying this, and meaning it, toward the end of the first interview, once I have a preliminary understanding. Some variants of this statement are: "Your problem is very longstanding and entrenched. I think I can help you make some progress on it, but it's going to take a long time," or "I think I can help you, but only if you also address your addiction directly by going to AA or some other program with a success rate in getting people off drugs," or "I think I can help you to understand and deal with the long-term problems with other people that have been the consequence of your phobias, but if you want to get some immediate relief from these terrifying attacks, you might try going first or simultaneously to a colleague of mine who specializes in the short-term treatment of phobic reactions," or " I am confident that I can help you, but only on the condition that you also see a psychiatrist about medication for your mood disorder," or "I can tell that you really have no hope that change is possible and are coming to me despite your sense of futility. I guess for a while I'll have to carry the hope for both of us."

Addressing Practicalities of the Therapy Contract

Time and Length of Meetings

There is no reason to leave unclear anything about the practical aspects of the professional contract. A part of the initial meeting, once the two parties have decided to work together, is finding a time they can get together. It is important that this be regular, unless the patient's schedule is erratic (this is true for some professional musicians and other performers, for example) and the therapist can accommodate a shifting meeting time without resentment. It is also important that the therapist not offer an appointment that he or she will begrudge keeping, such as very early in the morning or very late in the evening. I am careful in an initial interview to say something like, "I do forty-five-minute sessions. Sometimes I find myself letting the time run over a couple of minutes, especially if you're talking about something deeply involving, but in general, I'll end the session promptly." Occasionally, I have had patients ask me whether I would give them notice when there were five minutes left, and I usually consent to do so, though later, I look to understand the meaning of the request. My office has a clock in full view of the client, and behind such an entreaty usually lie some warded-off dependency needs and/or some hostility about the therapist's practice of ending the session on time.

Payment

Most beginning therapists find it hard to deal directly about money. I remember realizing, when I started practicing, that it was emotionally unimaginable to me to get paid for doing something I found so fascinating. Also, many clinicians undervalue themselves and what they offer, or feel anxiously competitive if they charge an amount comparable to that of their own therapist. But after a while, it becomes clear to even a self-abnegating practitioner that this is the way one earns one's living, and that the work, although endlessly rewarding, is also demanding and exhausting. Given that money is a reality of a professional relationship, it is important to be straightforward, unapologetic, and reasonable about it.

Such an attitude conveys that the therapist is appropriately concerned with his or her own welfare—a particularly good example to set for masochistic clients. It is also helpful to those who are inclined to test limits. I once treated a psychiatrist who later told me that one of the most therapeutic things I had done for him had occurred in our first meeting. When he asked me my fee, I asked him what he charged for a forty-five-minute session. When he told me, I said, "That would be fine for me, too." In fact, his fee was higher than my usual one, but I had a sense that he would privately disdain someone who charged less than he did (see Chapter Nine). In accounting for how this interchange had been therapeutic, he explained that he had needed to trust that I would take care of myself and not be manipulable, like his mother.

This is not my usual way of setting a fee. Ordinarily I simply say, "My fee is _____. Do you have any problem coming up with that?" If the patient makes a reasonable argument that my regular fee is a hardship, I am willing to slide somewhat, especially with people who want to come, and would profit from coming, more than once a week. (Because I enjoy treating patients who cannot afford the going rates for therapy, I also work four hours per week at quite low cost, and when I have such a low-fee opening, I put a less affluent person there and explain that I do a certain amount of low-cost work.) I also ask if the patient would prefer to pay after each session or by the month, and I add that if the person pays by the month, I would like to get the check by the middle of the following month, because I do not organize my finances such that I can carry bigger debts. I ask if the client wants a bill, or needs one for insurance purposes. If the bill is to be submitted to a third party, I ask that I be paid up front and have the reimbursement come to the patient, explaining that with this arrangement, whatever mistakes and postponements the insurance company personnel make—and in my experience, such errors are legion—the patient will be the one fighting with them for payment, not me.

I do not work with managed care companies. When a patient's benefits are with a managed care organization, I explain to him or her why I believe it is virtually impossible to do ethical therapy under managed care. Until fairly recently (lately, the word has been getting out), most clients have been shocked to learn that their confidentiality is compromised in such arrangements. They are also appalled that despite the fact that the managed care company marketed itself to their employer as providing a full range of psychotherapy services, in reality, all that is covered is short-term crisis intervention. The sleight of hand by which managed care organizations have devalued good mental health treatment and made it unavailable to everyone but the wealthy was accomplished by their promising to provide all the care that is "medically necessary" and then redefining medical necessity to exclude virtually all psychotherapy. I hope that by the time this book sees print there will be a strong public movement to replace this inherently flawed and ineffective system of "cost containment," in which money that used to pay for health care now goes into corporate profits.

A specific, practical problem of working with companies who have strong financial incentives for denying treatment is that when one argues that a client should continue in therapy because he or she is responding well to treatment, the response of the managers of care tends to be, "So you've accomplished a significant treatment goal. Time to terminate the patient." If, on the other hand, one states that the person is not doing well and needs more intensive or long-term therapy, the predictable response is, "Obviously you're not the right person for this patient. We'll end the treatment with you and recommend medication or another provider." Thus, termination is the treatment of choice whether the patient is improving or not. Once a client learns what will happen under a managed care policy, he or she usually prefers to pay out of pocket. I then negotiate a fee that the person can pay without shortchanging his or her family—and that I can accept without unduly depriving mine.

Cancellation Policy

I am in a minority among therapists in not having a cancellation policy. Most of my colleagues have some arrangement by which patients pay all or part of the hourly fee when they cancel with insufficient notice. A common rule is that if a client fails to let the treater know twenty-four hours ahead of their scheduled meeting, he or she will be charged for the session unless the two parties can agree on a time for a makeup session. At an extreme with respect to cancellation arrangements are the analysts who insist that their patients take vacations at the same time they do, and who otherwise charge them for time they take off from treatment, even for scheduled family vacations. These practices are sometimes quite central to the therapist's self-respect and therefore to his or her clinical functioning.

Cancellation policies follow the lead of Freud (1913), who argued that given the small number of individuals a full-time analyst treats, and the consequent importance to a therapist's income of each hour, it makes sense for the patient to "rent" a given appointment time and be responsible for it whether or not it is used. In other words, he suggested that undertaking therapy should be regarded as comparable to enrolling in an academic seminar: You can miss a class here or there, but you still have to pay for the whole course. From my perspective, the operative rule in choices about practice arrangements is that the therapist needs to protect against resenting the patient. It is very hard to have a sincere will to help a person by whom one feels demeaned or exploited.

Despite such considerations, I have been less influenced by Freud than by Frieda Fromm-Reichmann (1950) in these matters. Fromm-Reichmann argued that it is not customary in our society to charge for services not rendered and that in any case, a busy professional can make good use of the time freed up by cancellations. She felt that if a patient develops a pattern of canceling, there are ways to deal with it interpretively that will effectively address the behavior without imposing a sanction. An additional current consideration is that insurance companies typically do not pay for missed sessions (their executives seem to regard such policies as a scam, a rationalization for therapists' greed). As a result, for a patient using insurance, one has to keep track of the charges submitted for reimbursement alongside those that are not reimbursable. I find this kind of record keeping more onerous than just not charging. Also, my personal economy of scarcity involves time more than money; I am usually glad to have a free hour. Having said all this, I should note an exception to my general practice that applies to clients with significant psychopathy. With such patients, I lay down very strict rules from the outset about the client's financial responsibility for every session, whether the person comes or not.

One of my reasons for not charging for missed sessions is that I have a home office. When someone cancels, I am not stuck in a distant, rented suite with dead time on my hands and nowhere to go. I can always use the hour, if not to do something professional, then to do something domestic. I do charge for "no-shows," however, on the grounds that I am cooling my heels in my office, waiting. I do not describe my no-show policy during the first interview; I raise it if the situation comes up, and I implement it only after I have introduced the rule. Sophisticated patients often ask about a cancellation policy, and I am happy to give them my rationale if they express surprise at my lack of such a provision.

Diagnosis of Record

Some of my earliest training as a therapist was with rather authoritarian psychiatrists who promulgated the notion that no patient should ever be told his or her diagnosis. The stated justification for this position was that it might be upsetting and that it would contribute to the defense of intellectualization. I bridled at such ideas at the time, and I am even more negative about them now. The unstated agenda seems to me to be the preservation of the treater's superior power via private, inaccessible knowledge. Mystification has no place in psychotherapy (cf. Aron, 1996). Aside from the fact that anyone using insurance can find out his or her designated diagnosis by comparing the numbers on the bill with those in the DSM, it seems to me a matter of basic respect for the therapist to share the diagnosis, explain the basis for it, and discuss how the recommended treatment is appropriate to it. The practice of keeping a diagnosis from the patient also seems to me to reinforce the idea that emotional problems are somehow shameful, and that we should therefore convey information via euphemisms rather than in the language in which we really think about them.

Sometimes—and it is my impression that this is atypical, but it seems reasonable to me—I give the DSM to a client and show the person one or more diagnostic categories that pertain to the problems he or she came to work on, asking whether this label seems to describe accurately the person's complaints, or which of two possible diagnostic formulations is more nearly accurate. We thus make the official diagnosis together. Interesting information sometimes comes out of this process. I have had clients read a description of symptoms associated with the general category in which their psychopathology seems to fit, and then remark, "Oh, I forgot to tell you. I have that problem, too. I didn't think it was related." One woman whose mania I took months to diagnose correctly (because it manifested as rage, and it felt more like a borderline diatribe than mania) looked at the DSM once I suggested that a bipolar process might be going on with her, and on reading the list of symptoms, exclaimed, "I do have racing thoughts! And I go on shopping binges!" She had always been too angry in her manic states to mention these correlates of her mood.

Another woman who was very paranoid, and who I thought would feel criticized and arbitrarily pigeonholed if I unilaterally provided a diagnosis on her insurance form, asked me if she could look through the DSM (then the DSM-II [American Psychiatric Association, 1968]) when I told her I needed to submit a formal diagnosis for insurance purposes. I said that given the fact that she was trying to change certain lifelong patterns in treatment, the Personality Disorders section was probably the best place to look. She scrutinized the possibilities, and then announced with great satisfaction: "There I am: Paranoid Personality! Look, it says hypersensitive, rigid, suspicious, jealous, and tending to blame others! Sounds right to me." The fact that she (correctly) diagnosed herself made the process of looking at her paranoia a whole different enterprise than if I had given her the same label in a way she had felt was authoritarian.

I feel strongly that the diagnostic process should be as consensual as the therapy process. A professional may have greater expertise and general knowledge of psychology than patients do, but patients' specific knowledge about themselves is the material on which diagnoses are based. A recent essay by Anthony Hite (1996) on the "diagnostic alliance" has spoken for this attitude with particular persuasiveness. Again, there is nothing in our nosology that is impossible for a client to understand if the clinician explains what it is in ordinary speech. The pretense that the patient would not understand, or would be too upset by hearing the technical words that apply to his or her suffering, seems to me mainly a rationalization in the service of an illusory superiority.

I also treat the diagnostic issue as a kind of necessary evil, explaining that no one is an exact fit with any of the available categories, and that they are only the roughest approximations of very complex conditions. As I have written at length (McWilliams, 1994), I find DSM-type, descriptive psychiatric diagnosis to be both reductionistic and not particularly useful clinically, but if one needs to supply a third party with an official label, the DSM is the best and most universal taxonomy we have. Like most practitioners, I stop thinking in terms of prefabricated categories once I have a reliable feel for the unique psychology of any individual patient. I want the people who come to me for treatment to know from the beginning that this is my orientation: I want to know who they are, not what categories their symptoms match. Yet I do not withhold from them knowledge of the diagnosis of record.

Inviting Questions

At the end of an interview, I always ask if the client has any questions for me. More than half the people who come to me say at that point that they have nothing to ask; they feel good about the connection with me, and they look forward to our work together. Some people, out of either a sophistication about therapy or a good natural intuition, want to know nothing about me because they are interested in what they will project. Others have something very specific they want to address: What is my orientation? Where did I get my training? Have I had therapy myself? Do I have kids? Do I have any plans to move or retire? Am I in good health? What is my religious orientation? What do I think of deeply religious people? What are my politics? Do I think I can work without prejudice with someone of a minority sexual orientation? Am I specifically trained in trauma?

I respond to such concerns directly and economically. I feel it is a basic consumer right to get answers to questions that are a condition of hiring someone. While it is true that such queries always hint at deeper issues that might be fruitfully explored, an initial meeting does not seem to me the time to do it. The parties are still contracting for therapy; the employer (the patient) has not yet conferred upon the therapist the authority to begin interpreting. Anything significant to the client's psychology will reappear many times in the transference, whether or not it has been addressed realistically in an early meeting. Often, though, I handle such inquiries by saying something like, "I'll be glad to answer your question, but first, could you tell me why it's important to you to know that?" Because these early questions usually constitute tests (Weiss, 1993), it helps to know the client's thinking behind the request for information. Once the therapy is under way, I take a different attitude toward questions, examining them as they arise rather than just answering them.

Very rarely, someone will ask something in an initial meeting that feels too intrusive to me. For example, one or two prospective patients have asked me if I have ever had a lesbian relationship, and once I was asked if I had ever had an extramarital affair. In these instances, it seems to me important to be both honest and self-protective. What I tend to say is something like, "I can appreciate why that would be important for you to know, but I find myself feeling that my sexual life is too private for me to be comfortable answering that question. Are you afraid that if I have not had that experience I can't possibly understand you?" Honesty and intimate disclosure are not the same thing, and although the curiosity of a client may be frustrated by a limit-setting reply, there is often a simultaneous relief that the person in authority can be trusted to maintain professional boundaries.

Preparing the New Client to Give a History

Unless the interviewee has given a very full personal history in the initial session (something that characterizes therapists in training but almost no one else), I say at the end of the intake meeting something like the following:

> "So. We'll meet next Tuesday at nine o'clock. What I'd like to do then is to take a very complete history—your parents, what they were like, your childhood, the major influences on you, your sexual history, your work history, your prior therapy, your dreams, and so forth. This will give me a context in which to understand what you've talked about today. Then in the subsequent session, the ball will be more or less in your court again. You should come in and talk about whatever is foremost on your mind, and it will be my job to listen and help you make sense of your thoughts and feelings. Does that sound okay?"

I do this not only to reduce the anxiety that most people have about diving into an undefined and rather intimidating procedure, but also to encourage the client to start reflecting on his or her personal history and its contribution to the current problem. A lot of what happens in therapy goes on *between* the actual sessions. Organizing things this way also reduces my own anxiety about diving in before I have enough data to feel I can understand the person's difficulties.

Sharing a Dynamic Formulation with the Client

A full dynamic formulation goes way beyond a diagnostic label, in that it includes at least the eight topics I will cover in the chapters to come, but the same principles I just noted about sharing a DSM diagnosis apply to offering some of one's dynamic hypotheses for the client's consideration. It is important to keep one's inferences tentative, to be aware of their limitations, to check them out with the patient, and to engage mutually in an ongoing process of revision and elaboration of the ways the two parties understand the person's psychology. Although the sharing of a dynamic formulation should be mediated by timing and tact, clients have the right to know the therapist's working assumptions about the nature of their difficulties. In fact, the therapist's communication of his or her provisional conclusions about the origins and functions of the patient's problems typically becomes the cornerstone of the working alliance.

The sharing of the dynamic formulation also should contain some ideas about how the therapy, given this tentative understanding, will attempt to address the patient's problems. The clinician's ideas should be conveyed with a sense of hope and the expectation of a gratifying collaboration. Thus, the therapist might say something like the following:

> "So far, what hits me between the eyes about your depression is how many losses you've had that you haven't mourned, and how much your family discouraged your feeling sad by their criticism of your 'feeling sorry for yourself.' You might find you have some anger about that and other things that you haven't felt comfortable admitting, and if we can access the grief and the anger, your depression may lift. Also, there's some evidence for a depressive streak that's congenital in your family, and it doesn't sound like you've had anybody address that and help you cope by learning what situations tend to depress you and why. How does this sound to you?"

Here is another possible dynamic formulation, as communicated to the client:

> "It sounds like you are shy and sensitive by temperament, but it seems that no one in your family knew how to help you get braver around people. With the best intentions, they made things worse by forcing you into social situations, where you clutched. Because you had one after another failure socially, you began to think there was something very strange about you, and eventually you related only to yourself and your thoughts. You were lonely, but the idea of being close to someone terrified you. Then when your boss criticized you, you retreated even further into yourself, to the point that you were hearing voices. We need to work on getting you more comfortable with others, including me, and part of that will involve

looking at the things that you have believed make you so alien. Once we understand the meaning of some of your preoccupations, I think you'll find you're not so bizarre. In the meantime, if you're still hearing voices, you may want to consider seeing someone who will prescribe antipsychotic medications. Does that make sense to you?"

Educating the Patient about the Therapy Process

Just as a diagnosis and a dynamic formulation should not be withheld from a client, there is no reason for a therapist not to explain the rationale for any procedures he or she recommends (cf. Etchegoyen, 1991, on the democratic vs. authoritarian contract). Ordinary, nontechnical language is certainly adequate to express why one is interested in hearing the patient's dreams ("Very often I find that when nothing seems to be going on at the conscious level, a person's dreams will contain a lot of information about deeper preoccupations") or free associations ("The more freely you can talk, the better I can understand you; if you find yourself censoring anything, try to talk about it anyway, or at least tell me that you are finding it hard to talk about something") or memories ("The first step to resolving a problem is often understanding where it came from").

The same thing applies to clinical interest in the patient's reactions to the therapist. Most clients are somewhat taken aback by being asked what they are thinking and feeling about the practitioner; this was not what they expected to be talking about. They wonder if the therapist is asking out of insecurity or vanity or a need to feel reassured. Early in therapy, if I notice that a person seems uncomfortable with my asking how he or she is feeling toward me, I will say something like the following:

"I know it's strange to be asked to be so direct, and it must feel awkward, especially when some of your responses to me are negative. But in a way, therapy is a microcosm, a chance to study a relationship at close range, and by investigating what happens between you and me, we have an opportunity to scrutinize some emotional things that may happen to you elsewhere, things no one talks about in social situations. You may find yourself feeling toward me the way you feel or have felt toward other people, and our comprehension of that should be very useful in your efforts to understand yourself and change."

This matter-of-fact, educative style applies also to more esoteric aspects of some therapies, including the famous analytic couch. There is nothing mysterious about the couch. I tell people that its utility was discovered accidentally by Freud, who had people lie down and look away from him because he got sick of being stared at all day. I go on to say that like a lot of serendipitous discoveries, analysts have learned that it has another, much more important effect. It not only allows the patient to relax, it also takes the therapist out of eye contact. Without being able to see the clinician's face, the client may notice that he or she has ideas about what the therapist is thinking or feeling that never came to mind before. I comment that, very often, people carry around a lot of unconscious apprehensions about what other people's reactions to them will be, and they learn to scan others' faces and disconfirm their fears before they even know they have them. The patient's use of the couch will bring such anxieties into awareness. I also say that I like to work using the couch because, like Freud, I find it tiring to be scanned, and I enjoy sitting back, not making eye contact, and thinking about how the client's words are stirring up my own associations.

These communications may all be considered part of the development of a working alliance. Greenson (1967, p. 196) gave a memorable example of this kind of education of a man who had gone through a long previous psychoanalysis without ever having been told the rationale for various analytic procedures. While obtaining a history, Greenson asked him his middle name. The patient, who had a pathologically compliant personality, thought he should free associate and answered, "Raskonikrov." This man was obeying what he regarded as the "rule" of free association, but he failed to get the whole point of the analytic enterprise. Greenson goes on to talk about how fruitless psychotherapy is in the absence of a working alliance in which both parties understand what is required of them, and why. In fact, a relationship without such a basis is a caricature of therapy.

CONCLUDING COMMENTS

There is an apocryphal story about D. W. Winnicott, the great British object relations theorist, that applies to the general tone of interviewing and treatment. I do not remember who told it to me, but here is the gist: Winnicott was once asked what his rules for interpreting were. He answered, "I interpret for two reasons. One, to let the patient know that I am awake, and two, to let the patient know I can be wrong." Aside from being funny, there is great wisdom in this quip. If the therapist is doing his or her job properly, the client will be repeatedly correcting and revising the formulations that the therapist offers. The realization that the therapist is frequently wrong is one of the great therapeutic revelations. Patients will forgive almost anything except arrogance, and they are grateful for models of nondefensiveness. I recently asked a friend of mine how his analysis was going. "Great!" he replied. "He admits when he makes a mistake!"

On the topic of one's inevitable limitations and errors, I want to be sure the reader knows that my thinking about each of the issues I will address in the following chapters is not the kind of mental reflection I do in a typical clinical session. I am very good at organizing information once I have assimilated it, but the nature of a clinical interview—especially an intake interview—involves a kind of disorganized not knowing. As is evident in the previous examples, the formulations one floats to a client are neither so elegant nor so complex that they would require vast psychoanalytic knowledge to make. Even if I were capable of constructing a truly comprehensive formulation during the first interview, it would not be useful for the patient, who comes not to be wowed by the therapist's erudition but to see if there is a human being out there who wants to understand and has sufficient training to help.

I recently did an intake interview with a psychologist, a woman with an extensive background in the helping professions. I asked why she had chosen me as a therapist. Her reply was, "Because I hate you." I asked for some elaboration. "When I read your book," she said, "I got so angry that you knew all that stuff, and I'd been practicing for years and didn't know a lot of it. So I hated you. I want to get what you have." What I have is a capacity to take dense and sometimes preverbal material and make sense of it in the categories of psychoanalytic theories as I understand them. I am grateful for this capacity, and over the years I have come to appreciate it in myself and realize that it represents a personal synthesis of sorts that is not too common. But it operates only in retrospect, not in the immediacy of clinical contact, where I can be completely baffled and inarticulate. This patient who hates me will soon find that for many months, she will understand herself a lot better than I do, because whatever her blind spots turn out to be, she has already spent many years thinking about herself and her unique psychology. Similarly, I hope my readers understand that their skill or lack thereof at reeling off concepts post hoc has very little to do with whether they are good therapists in the heat of the clinical moment.

SUMMARY

I have tried here to give readers a feel for the process of clinical evaluation. With some caveats about its possible inapplicability to the situations of many therapists, I have given details of and rationales for my own practices during intake interviews, including my efforts to make a safe connection, to minimize anxiety, to elicit the client's reaction to me, to convey understanding, to assess reactions to my clinical hypotheses, to impart hope, and to address the practicalities of the therapy contract. These latter matters include issues of time, payment, cancellation, diagnosis of record, questions, and preparation for history taking. I have further discussed the importance of sharing the tentative dynamic formulation and doing some straightforward education of the client about any puzzling aspects of the recommended treatment. Finally, despite the fact that the following chapter topics represent central questions that analytic practitioners are trying to answer so that they can orient treatment properly, I have emphasized how during an intake interview one cannot reasonably expect to feel that everything has fallen into place and that one has a comprehensive understanding of the patient.

CHAPTER THREE

Assessing What Cannot Be Changed

THERAPISTS have not written much about unchangeable aspects of people's individual psychologies. When we work with someone in psychotherapy, we focus on what *can* be changed because we are hired as agents of change. Nonetheless, for many reasons, we need to acknowledge and appreciate the significance of those aspects of a person's situation that are not amenable to therapeutic influence. A person's basic temperament is one thing that therapy does not change, and numerous other fixed aspects of people's individual psychologies also set limits on, and provide a context for, our therapeutic efforts. These include, but are not limited to, other genetic givens, such as dyslexia or a vulnerability to bipolar illness; irreversible consequences to the brain of physical trauma, toxicity, or infection; and chronic physical illness or body compromise of any kind. Of a different order but still important to appreciate in any overall formulation of a person's psychological situation are those facts of life that are individually unchangeable for that person, facts that come under the colloquial heading of "harsh realities," such as being incarcerated, being a member of a visible minority group, or having an autistic child.

Most writing on psychotherapy stresses the goal of change: change in behavior, mood, habits of defense, developmental preoccupations, and so forth. A less frequently emphasized aspect of psychotherapy is adaptation to those features of life that cannot be changed, including the client's development of strategies that compensate for unchangeable realities. The adaptation process involves the overcoming of denial, the transformation of magical ideas into mourning and coping, and the substitution of realistic explanations for pathogenic beliefs. It opens the door to better, more authentic relationships, based on the acceptance of one's immutable attributes. Of course, this is a profound kind of change in itself.

Although coming to terms with something that cannot be changed may seem less exciting as a therapeutic goal than exorcizing one's dispensable neurotic demons, the adaptive process is crucial to human well-being. No one who has been through it underestimates its importance. A man with a deep, genetically influenced susceptibility to depression cannot expect ever to be free of depressive episodes, yet he can learn to react to them with self-acceptance rather than self-hatred, to substitute appropriate medication for either substance abuse or self-denying bravado, and to tell those who love him what he is going through rather than lapsing into inarticulate, exasperating withdrawal. These are not trivial accomplishments, as anyone with a depressive history can attest.

It is critical to the success of any therapy to have reasonable goals. A dynamic formulation should, among other things, establish in the clinician's mind a clarity about what is feasible and what is not. The therapist's sharing with the patient his or her tentative hypotheses about what will be possible sets the stage for both parties' being able to measure their progress against realistic expectations. This communication begins a mourning process for the client, who has inevitably come to therapy with some residual infantile hopes for magical transformation. It models ego strength, in that the therapist is seen as capable of naming very upsetting aspects of reality without collapsing into a sense of futility in the face of what has been named. It conveys empathy. It also protects against the demoralization and loss of self-esteem in both parties, in that pursuing the unattainable inevitably creates shame about failure.

In this chapter I discuss clinical implications of several types of unchangeable realities, including (1) temperament, (2) genetic, congenital, and medical conditions with direct psychological effects, (3) irreversible brain conditions caused by trauma, illness, or toxicity, (4) unalterable features of the body, including chronic physical illness, (5) unalterable external circumstances, and (6) personal history. This list is probably not exhaustive, as life has a way of throwing one after another immovable obstacle in anyone's path, but I hope it is extensive enough to make what I think of as an essential clinical point.

TEMPERAMENT

Academic psychologists have come a long way from the radically behavioristic and naively pragmatic era in which John Watson could boast, "Give me a dozen healthy infants . . . and I'll guarantee to take any one at random and train him to become any type of specialist I might select—doctor, lawyer, artist, merchant-chief and, yes, even beggar-man and thief, regardless of his talents, penchants, tendencies, abilities, vocation, and race of his ancestors" (1925, p. 82). Beginning roughly in midcentury with the careful work of researchers like Sybille Escalona (1968) and Thomas, Chess, and Birch (1968), and culminating recently in Kagan's (1994) comprehensive analysis, researchers have confronted and described the limitations that basic temperament imposes on any individual person. A generation of developmental scholarship has convincingly demonstrated that human beings are anything but blank slates at birth. From shyness to stimulation seeking, we know that people's attributes are genetically influenced and cannot be seen as sheerly the result of their upbringing. The fact that therapists pay a lot of attention to people's nurture rather than nature reflects the fact that this is the part of one's heritage that could have been different, that could have led to different consequences that now can be imagined and pursued. This therapeutic focus on environment should not be misunderstood as minimizing the importance of genetic endowment.

One common clinical experience in which an appreciation of the importance of temperament takes on special significance involves working with someone who was adopted. An individual can be nurtured from earliest infancy on by an unambiguously loving family and still feel profoundly alienated and misunderstood because there is no one in the adoptive family system that viscerally understands his or her basic temperament. It is natural for adoptive parents to minimize the "differentness" of the child they bring up as their own, and to hope that their love for that child will be received emotionally as no different from the love of biological parents. Because of such hopes, there is often a forbidden emotional territory in an adoptive family, a prohibition on the child's expressing feelings of pain and isolation, or articulating the ways in which he or she seems temperamentally out of sync with other family members.

The significance of this for clinical practice is that by focusing on temperament and its vast implications, a clinician can help an adopted client to confront, examine, and reject the painful conclusions he or she has typically drawn from a childhood experience of ineffable emotional estrangement. Typically, the youngster whose temperamental proclivities are alien and problematic to his or her parents develops the conviction that there is just something "wrong" with the self. Such inferences in adoptees are usually connected to the fantasy that "It is because of what is wrong with me that my natural parents rejected me." Psychotherapy can transform such pathogenic beliefs into realistic appreciation of the facts of a client's history. Adoption is an inherently arbitrary process whose nature defies the child's natural wish for fairness. "The adoption agency could have sold me to anyone," one of my patients mused. Appreciating this stark fact of life helped him to grieve over the fact that, in unfair contrast to children living with their biological parents, he had been deprived of caretakers whose rhythms and intensities were more likely to have mirrored his own. His sense of inner shame and badness thus shifted toward resignation about a particular personal misfortune.

Adoptees are not the only people who feel temperamentally isolated in their families of origin. Genetic endowment being somewhat accidental, individuals can inherit a temperament that neither of their parents recognizes as familiar, or (perhaps more ominously) can inherit one that reminds a mother or father of a hated relative. Intense children whose parents are placid typically get told that there is something wrong with them for "overreacting" to everything. Shy children of sociophilic parents get pushed aggressively at people they are not yet ready to approach. High-activity offspring of couch potatoes inspire anything from mild criticism to physical abuse. Speaking of which, I have yet to meet an adult with a severely colicky infant who did not observe spontaneously that he or she now knew how a sleep-deprived, exhausted parent could hit a defenseless infant. The knowledge that one was colicky and difficult can replace a client's prior conclusion that he or she was simply "bad." Understanding the plain facts of a situation tends to take the stigma out of it.

Although temperament cannot be changed, its behavioral expression can be modified. Research with constitutionally shy and socially phobic children, for example, has led to the development of specific, step-by-step interventions that gradually allow them to increase their range of comfort in dealing with people (Rapee, 1998). There is also a popular but scholarly literature on shyness (e.g., Zimbardo, 1990) that can provide enormous enlightenment and comfort to shy people and their families. Greenspan's (1996) book on "the challenging child" has been a godsend to parents with a temperamentally difficult youngster. This is true for numerous other conditions with a genetic component as well. For example, many adults coping with previously undiagnosed attention deficit disorder have found both solace and practical help in the aptly titled *You Mean I'm Not Lazy, Crazy, or Stupid?!* (Kelly & Ramundo, 1995).

GENETIC, CONGENITAL, AND MEDICAL CONDITIONS WITH DIRECT PSYCHOLOGICAL EFFECTS

When supervising or consulting on the work of other therapists, I am often struck by the extent to which physically limiting conditions are ignored or minimized—even by practitioners with medical backgrounds, who have presumably more training in diagnostic evaluation for what was until recently called organicity.* For example, one otherwise capable student of mine was perplexed by why an "obsessive–compulsive" Native American boy was not responding well to treatment. It turned out she was ignoring compelling evidence that the child's main difficulties involved the long-term effects of fetal alcohol syndrome. It is understandable that a therapist would wish that a child's condition were more treatable and had a better prognosis. But by denying the actual diagnostic state of affairs, this well-meaning clinician was involving the child in an approach that was doomed to fail and was depriving him of the help that does exist, even though it comes more under the heading of "management" than "therapy" for people with his disability.

A related question that is often missed in an intake interview is whether the client's psychological problems may represent the expression of a physical illness. Not only does depression tend to reduce the power of the immune system, so that depressed people get sick more than nondepressed ones, but the converse is also true: Being sick makes people depressed. But even beyond this general point, there are many diseases with well-established psychological correlates. These include, for example, Lyme disease, diabetes mellitus, hyperthyroidism, myasthenia gravis, multiple sclerosis, pernicious anemia, rheumatoid arthritis, and many others. I strongly recommend that both medical and nonmedical therapists obtain James Morrison's (1997) useful guide, *When Psychological Problems Mask Medical Disorders*, for help in disentangling somatic and psychological issues.

One of my concerns about the current climate in which mental health services are delivered is that third-party pressures for the briefest treatment incline clinicians not to "waste time" with careful formula-

---

*In the DSM-IV, the term "organic" has been replaced by "due to a general medical condition," because recent research has demonstrated the physical bases for various psychopathologies that were once considered "functional." In other words, there are organic contributants to many psychopathologies that we used to think of as strictly expressions of individual experience.

tion, especially if the diagnostic process involves something extra, like a neurological consultation. Time is much more seriously wasted if a patient is being "treated" for something other than his or her primary malady. Particularly in cases where a client presents odd symptomatology that does not fall easily into any of the more common syndrome categorizations, taking a careful developmental history is critical. Such investigations sometimes reveal previously ignored facts such as oxygen deprivation at birth, maternal abuse of substances during pregnancy, or the possible effects of prescribed medications on a person's fetal development. It is a serious mistake to conclude reflexively, for example, that a woman who reports early masculine-like behaviors has identified with her father. One possibility—among many—is that she was affected by prenatal androgens (Money, 1988). The way the therapist should respond to her reports of her inclinations would be significantly different if the causes of her childhood demeanor were primarily hormonal rather than experiential.

Similarly, it has radically affected treatment that we are beginning to have a body of well-controlled research on the biological substrates for conditions such as the schizophrenias and the mood disorders. Progress in psychopharmacology has meant enormous gains in the emotional welfare of some people who could never have been helped before. Although controversy still rages over psychopharmacological versus psychotherapeutic treatment (much complicated by the obvious financial interests of drug companies and the insurance industry in recommending medication rather than talk therapy), a preponderance of research suggests that especially for seriously disturbed individuals, both are critical. Despite the fact that practitioners like me, who do the psychotherapy part, can frequently be heard lamenting the contemporary overreliance on drugs and underreliance on therapy, it is still true that the existence of medications such as mood stabilizers, antidepressants, and antipsychotic drugs have made a decent life possible for many people who previously simply suffered and died. For an interviewer to miss, for example, the evidence that a person's hypersexuality expresses a pharmacologically treatable manic condition is to do a significant disservice to the client.

IRREVERSIBLE CONSEQUENCES OF HEAD TRAUMA, ILLNESS, AND TOXICITY

I remember vividly a case I was assigned early in my training, a seventeen-year-old young man who went into frightening rages. He had been referred to the mental health center where I worked because he had tried to run down his high school principal with his car. When I presented the case to the treatment team, I commented that he had seemed to relate to me frankly and with sincere upset about his explosiveness, and that I thought more was going on than some kind of general antisocial orientation. The psychiatrist leading the discussion took an immediately disdainful position and made an example of me as a naive young therapist who had been a sitting duck for an adolescent con artist. Fortunately, I was able to convey my impressions of this client to a more respectful person in authority who was willing to have the boy seen by a neurologist. It turned out that he had a lesion in the temporal lobe, and that his rage outbursts could be substantially reduced by medications that control epilepsy. If no one had been willing to listen to me at that point, a fate that beginning therapists confront all too often, this earnest, confused, and dangerous youngster would probably have become a casualty of the juvenile justice system.

Both medical and nonmedical therapists often fail to take the kind of history that will illuminate possible brain pathology. The book (Sacks, 1990) and movie *Awakenings* depicted poignantly the experience of a whole group of mental patients whose commonalities were only appreciated and subjected to condition-specific treatment when a particularly conscientious professional, insistent upon researching their histories, learned that all of them had had encephalitis lethargica in the "sleeping sickness" epidemic of 1917. (The tragedy of the story is that the successful treatment with the drug L-Dopa of the comatose aftereffects of sleeping sickness quickly created a nightmare of side effects that eventually became unbearable for the patients so afflicted.)

I knew a man who had had encephalitis during the 1917 epidemic and seemed to have completely recovered, despite having been in a coma for several weeks at age eleven. The only thing in his manner that overtly suggested any possibility of residual brain damage was a very slight oddness to his gait. In addition, during an army induction physical exam, a doctor who noticed that his pupils dilated unevenly had once greatly offended him by asking if he had ever had syphilis. To all external appearances, this man was perfectly normal. He had a good marriage, healthy and happy children, and a very responsible job. He did, however, become quite disorganized if certain basic routines were disrupted, and he tended to go into moralistic rages when upset. He also had no capacity for ambivalence: He either liked a person or subjected him or her to complete rejection. This intolerance of grey areas in human relationships might have suggested a borderline personality disorder characterized by the defense mechanism of splitting, except that nothing else about him seemed borderline.

This man's organic vulnerability became a serious problem only when his wife died of cancer. He became catastrophically upset and explosive. Anyone treating this bereaved and overwhelmed father could easily have missed the evidence of brain damage and disorganized him even further by encouraging him mainly in an emotionally cathartic direction. For decades, we have known about the critical role of structure and routine in the lives of brain-damaged people (Goldstein, 1942), and in conformance with the implications of this literature, what was eventually most helpful to this man and his family was a therapist's combination of reestablishing routines and educating his children about how to respond helpfully to his outbursts. Critical to her ability to do this was, of course, an attitude toward case formulation that did not minimize the possibility of brain dysfunction even in ostensibly functional subjects.

Research in the 1980s (Lewis, Pincus, Feldman, Jackson, & Bard, 1986; Lewis et al., 1988) with condemned criminals found that a startling percentage had sustained permanent head trauma. Even though the effects of such injury are not always treatable, the lumping together, either in research projects or in treatment programs, of people whose destructiveness results from brain pathology with those who are characterologically psychopathic in the absence of demonstrable physical damage can only lead to bad research and bad intervention. And occasionally, as with the angry young man who had a lesion of the temporal lobe, effective treatment is available once the etiology is clear.

One should also pursue in an interview the implications of any evidence that a person has a significant history of substance abuse. One woman I worked with had taken a near-fatal overdose of cocaine in her twenties, after a long period of regular use. She earnestly believed that this experience had done irreversible damage to her mental agility, and, in fact, her current measured IQ, though well over 100, was more than a standard deviation lower than she had tested before the overdose. It was critical to her comfort in therapy with me that I take seriously her belief that in her addiction she had done herself irreparable harm. Given considerable literature suggesting long-term cognitive impairment in cocaine-dependent people (reviewed in Huang & Nunes, 1995), I was inclined to believe that she had been damaged intellectually.

Other possible outcomes of substance abuse include Marchiafava–Bignami disease, which may present with personality changes in long-term alcoholics, the nutrient-deficiency-related illnesses such as Korsakoff's syndrome in alcoholics (Huang & Nunes, 1995), and memory problems and a loss of the capacity to concentrate in people who have taken marijuana regularly for years (Schwartz, 1991). There are probably many other subtler and more idiosyncratic outcomes of chemical assault on the brain that we have yet to understand and document. My point is that facing with the patient the fact that there may be some physiological limits to his or her mental capacities, limits set by prior drug abuse, is a necessary condition of realistic therapy.

UNCHANGEABLE PHYSICAL REALITIES

A person's sense of the integrity of his or her body is a natural basis of self-esteem and emotional health. In *The Ego and the Id*, Freud (1923) commented on how the earliest sense of ego or self is a "body ego," the physical sensation of the corporeality of the self and an understanding of its possibilities and limitations. The popularity of this phrase among analysts, even though Freud used it only once, suggests that the concept has widespread intuitive appeal. When someone's bodily integrity is compromised by accident, victimization, or illness, mourning is necessary if depression is to be avoided. When a therapist works with someone with a disability or chronic illness, a recognition of the significance of that factor is critical to the development of the therapeutic relationship. I do not mean that the therapist should necessarily extend sympathy, as patients in tragic circumstances are often offended to be on the receiving end of what they experience as a demeaning kind of pity, but the therapist must find a way to convey appreciation of the far-reaching consequences of the client's condition.

Sometimes the challenge for the therapist is to help the patient with the denial by which so many people handle their physical limitations. Once I took a long history from a man, an accomplished physician, in which we covered just about every aspect of his background, current situation, and interests. At the end of the session I asked, "Is there anything that I haven't asked about you or that you haven't volunteered that would be important for me to know?" "Well, I do have multiple sclerosis," he casually replied, "but it's no big deal." While it is true that an optimistic attitude about debility is probably an asset to physical health, the obliteration of reality to retain a false optimism is doubtless its enemy. It became clear that the first thing I should try to understand about this man was his need to minimize the implications of his having a serious chronic illness. Denial is maladaptive to making self-protective medical decisions.

A breast cancer patient whose optimistic problem-solving tendencies propel her into joining a support group where she can learn ways to fight her illness is much better off than the woman who denies that her cancer can recur and avoids monthly breast self-examinations so that her denial will not be threatened. In one famous study of breast cancer patients (Spiegel, Bloom, Kraemer, & Gottheil, 1989), members of a support group for women with advanced malignancies and grave prognoses lived an average of eighteen months longer than similar breast cancer patients without such a group. This is an eye-opening finding, considering both the usual life expectancy for late-stage carcinomas and the fact that these patients were recurrently dealing with the deaths of their sister group members, something that intuitively many of us would consider too stressful to be healthy. One conclusion I draw from these data is that even the most painful truths are the ally of adaptation.

It is a condition of contemporary life that most therapists see people with HIV infection and AIDS, another poignant circumstance in which unchangeable facts of life dwarf other aspects of an individual's psychology. There is beginning to be a good literature available to therapists struggling with patients for whom chronic and possibly terminal illness is the main issue (see, e.g., Goodheart & Lansing, 1997, on psychotherapeutic interventions with patients who have chronic disease of any kind, and Blechner's [1997] edited volume of essays on therapy with people who have AIDS and HIV). Because it will help the therapist understand some of the possible deeper meanings of the client's suffering, it is still important to take a full history when someone presents with an overwhelming harsh reality like a devastating disease, but one should be careful to convey that whatever the personal background, coping with the illness is the central task of the individual's current life.

Unchangeable facts of the body also include visible mutilations or disfigurements. One woman I worked with who had a congenital facial deformity spent most of her sessions with me talking about her anger at the way people both averted their eyes from her and then tried to study her physiognomy when they thought she was not looking. When she sensed me doing the same thing, she finally got a chance to tell someone off directly about it. This was a little hard for me to tolerate, as it usually is when patients experience me as hurting them in just the ways that the rest of the world has always done, but it turned out to be highly therapeutic for her. Her relief in the opportunity to be honest about her rage and misery was palpable. Her parents, who had spent considerable money on cosmetic surgery that had diminished the most off-putting aspects of her appearance, needed to feel she was grateful and happy with the result, and her lover, a woman she had lived with for several years, was invested in trying to persuade her that the irregularity of her features was hardly noticeable.

Although this woman had ostensibly come to therapy to deal with relationship problems with her partner, it became quickly clear that her prior need was to have a place where she could finally talk about her disfigurement and its profound implications. This concern turned out to be anything but independent of the interpersonal problems she was having, in that she believed at some level that she was so ugly that no one could love her. She had long ago concluded that anyone who seemed to be attracted to someone as deformed as she was must be either stupid, crazy, or possessed of some hidden agenda she would have to ferret out. Because she could not accept without suspicion any indications of her partner's genuine caring, she was treating her generosity and concern with rejection or disdain. The relationship issues sorted themselves out fairly well once the unconscious meanings and strategies about her appearance had been addressed in the transference with me.

UNCHANGEABLE LIFE CIRCUMSTANCES

The theme of coming to terms with unalterable limitations is an old one in psychoanalytic writing. Even people who are perfectly "normal" must mourn and renounce aims that cannot be realized, and in the ordinary course of development, most of us do this more or less successfully. Psychoanalytic experience suggests that we all harbor irrational desires to be simultaneously child and adult, male and female, gay and straight, old and young, independent and dependent; we all want to live forever. Freud (1940) emphasized as stubbornly problematic two universal infantile strivings that tend to remain unconscious (thereby making trouble): the wish of women to be male as well as female (penis envy), and the wish of heterosexual men for some homosexual attachment. In a society as patriarchal as turn-of-the-century Vienna, it is not surprising that disowned wishes to be male or to be erotically connected with males tended to surface in people's analyses. Later psychoanalytic writers (e.g., Bettelheim, 1954) felt that Freud's blind spots about his own psychology had led him to underestimate even deeper and more energetically disowned wishes in men, wishes that transcend any particular cultural context; namely, to be female and able to bear children (parturition envy).

A central idea about psychotherapy early in the twentieth century was that the patient should be helped to be conscious of irrational but powerful longings and to come to terms with the impossibility of gratifying them. The acknowledgment and gradual relinquishment of unrealizable wishes—in other words, a nontraumatic grieving process—would ideally replace the ways in which unconscious desires had previously been handled (e.g., in the case of unconscious wishes to be the other gender, by acting out hostility toward members of the opposite sex, by sexual inhibition, by symptoms that kept painful longings out of consciousness, by promiscuity whose underlying impetus was the "possessing" of the other). The conscious renunciation of futile strivings would set people free to spend more psychological energy on what was realistically achievable and gratifying.

It is still an ideal of psychoanalytic education that at least the practitioners of analysis should have become acquainted with their deepest, most infantile and prelogical desires and have made their peace with them. In analytic training, it is assumed that analysts cannot listen to clients nondefensively if they have not confronted all their own unrealizable longings and worked through their defenses against noticing and mourning them. The idea that therapy should bring irrational wishes and beliefs into awareness so that they can be examined, renounced, and replaced with more realistic and attainable aims—the classical objectives of making the unconscious conscious and replacing id with ego—has never disappeared from the psychodynamic therapy tradition, even though contemporary analysts tend to stress other aspects of the therapy process more. (Good ideas seldom die; they just resurface in other language. Some contemporary cognitive-behavioral practitioners are strikingly like the early analysts in their central emphasis on pointing out irrational beliefs and coaching clients to consider alternatives.)

In the contemporary practice of psychotherapy, it is a lucky clinician who has a patient who is motivated enough—and financially endowed enough—to pursue the intensive analysis that will address primal longings in a deep way. But we all see people who have more prosaic, less irrational, less deeply unconscious issues to grieve and who need to talk to someone who will let that process happen without trying to cheer them up, distract them, join their denial, or minimize their pain. Examples of clients who need therapists to appreciate their unalterable circumstances without getting defensive are people in stigmatized minority groups, people who are legally incarcerated, people with damaged children or failing parents or other consuming dependents, people who have lost jobs and are confronting an indifferent economic environment, and people in financial distress that does not admit of a prompt remedy. Just as Freud's female patients could not solve their problems by unconsciously appropriating maleness, contemporary clients with stubborn realities cannot handle them effectively by a combination of denial and magical thinking.

I am stressing these things in a book about case formulation because although one might think it self-evident that therapists should give the patient a forum for venting feelings about stark facts of life, I have frequently seen practitioners skirt just such issues. Critical to a client's initial willingness to work with a particular therapist is his or her feeling that the therapist does not flinch from talking about the ruthless realities the person faces. Perhaps avoidant clinicians feel that unless the problem is something they can actively alleviate, they might as well evade it. Or perhaps they feel burdened and compromised by the knowledge that they cannot extend honest empathy into these areas because there is nothing comparable in their own lives. I suspect that among other motives, we all fear calling attention to realms in which clients will, if given a chance, express frank envy and hatred over the therapist's comparative good fortune, thereby activating our survivor guilt (Lifton, 1968) and exposing our inability to make reparation.

The literature on working with clients in racial and ethnic minorities (e.g., Boyd-Franklin, 1989; Sue & Sue, 1990) consistently urges practitioners to encourage patients to discuss their feelings about race and ethnicity and, specifically, the differences between them and their therapists. That this point needs to be made over and over suggests that there are powerful resistances in therapists to forthrightness about issues of diversity. I have worked with otherwise sophisticated Caucasian supervisees who regularly "forget" to ask their African-American clients how they feel about having a white therapist. I used to feel impatient with them, but recently I ran into the same inhibition in myself in an initial interview with a person of color who was not spontaneously bringing up any concerns about our racial difference. There is a lot of socialization about what it is polite or impolite to mention that goes against good clinical practice, and doubtless a lot of unconscious racism and ethnocentrism that also militates against the candor in which psychotherapy must be conducted. ("This is psychoanalysis, not a tea party," one of my supervisors told me in response to my reluctance to ask an Asian patient directly how she felt about working with someone whose background was so different from her own.)

Similar difficulties may characterize heterosexual therapists working with gay, lesbian, and bisexual patients. Several psychoanalytic writers have recently critiqued how sexually straight therapists working with young and closeted gay patients are apt to understand such clients as sexually confused or undecided rather than to face clear evidence that they are predominantly homosexual (e.g., Frommer, 1995; Lesser, 1995). In other words, they are complicit with the patient's reluctance to acknowledge a distressing reality, both because they assume the patient is more like them than is true, and because they want to avoid witnessing the suffering of someone who must now mourn the fact that his or her particular psychology makes a mainstream lifestyle impossible. With gay and lesbian clients who have an established sexual identity, especially with those who are "out," heterosexual therapists often commit the converse error: In the rush to show their lack of antihomosexual bias, they unwittingly convey to clients of differing sexual orientation that they do not think it appropriate for them to be suffering in any way about something as unremarkable as homosexuality. This defensively "counterhomophobic" stance (McWilliams, 1996) can easily deter a patient from expressing pain related to sexual orientation or discussing the burdens of being in a socially marginal group. It can also support any denial the client may be using about the more problematic and distressing implications of his or her erotic makeup, such as increased risk of AIDS, dangers of persecution, and complications attending the wish to have children.

Patients typically generate fantasies about the therapist's freedom from cruel limitation. In part, this represents a realistic appraisal of the fact that the therapist is employed, is generally a member of the majority culture, may appear free of physical handicaps, and tends to behave as if most problems are at least addressable, if not solvable. In part it is wishful: People hope to evade their own suffering by identification with someone who presumably "has it all together." While most of us enjoy idealization, it does not come without the price tag of the patient's contrasting demoralization. Therefore, it is clinically advisable to assess the ways in which any individual client feels inferior or at a disadvantage compared to the therapist and to explore what that means for the person. Of course, this has to be done with tact, and with a sensitivity to the possibility of the client's feeling exposed and humiliated. In this process, it is important that the therapist be open to admitting that there are areas where his or her life is easier than the client's and also that there are areas where the client has the edge.

PERSONAL HISTORY

One other obvious but perhaps insufficiently explicated region in the category of "unchangeable" is anyone's personal history. Again, this seems perhaps too self-evident to mention, and yet numerous problems in psychotherapy can derive from patients' reluctance to accept the facts that nothing can change what has happened to them and that no one will hurry to compensate them for their undeserved suffering of prior years. Moreover, human sympathy and grandiosity being what they are, therapists are chronically tempted to imply that they can undo the damage of the past—as opposed to helping patients acknowledge it and move on anyway. Just as a woman who was malnourished in childhood cannot by eating properly as an adult undo all the harm her body has endured, a person who was psychologically abused in childhood cannot expect to be free of emotional scars. But what he or she *can* expect is not insignificant.

People frequently try to avoid mourning historical facts by clinging relentlessly to a defense of entitlement; that is, they feel that given the unfairness in their individual backgrounds, life (including the therapist) owes them reparation. Sometimes, especially among patients with particularly terrible histories, it takes months or years for them to assimilate the fact that therapy is not about airing grievances and getting others to make restitution but about solving their current problems. Therapists who join in their patients' fantasies about getting perpetrators to compensate for their historical crimes are courting disaster. In fact, along with Frawley-O'Dea (1996), I would argue that the whole false memory syndrome movement that has so troubled those of us working with trauma victims would not have arisen if some therapists had not joined their patients' resistance to mourning what cannot be changed and encouraged them to sue those they remembered as having molested them. It may be true in a legal sense that criminals should be held responsible for their crimes, but in psychotherapy, the important message for patients to get is that the power to change their lives inheres within them, unrelated to whether their childhood mistreaters admit to responsibility for their traumatization. When working with someone who has succeeded in getting a childhood abuser to confess the crime and try to make reparation, one is still struck by the fact that even though it reassures the patient that he or she was not "crazy" in remembering the abuse (not an inconsequential result but not all the patient hopes for), there is no sudden alleviation of its legacy of misery. In fact, there is usually a painful depressive reaction to the fact that even though the villain has confessed, the damage has been done and cannot be undone. The initial emotional reaction most of us have to a person's retrospective admission of culpability—for example, when a recovering alcoholic father apologizes to an adult child for the harm caused to him or her by his drinking—is usually a grudging "Too little, too late."

It is critical even in the briefest therapeutic intervention for a clinician to "get" what someone wants to avoid facing about the consequences of his or her personal background. The patient will profit in direct proportion to the degree to which the therapist can facilitate mourning, either immediately or eventually, when the client reflects on the therapeutic interaction. It is usually something of a revelation to patients, especially younger ones, that even if their parents were able at this point to change, they themselves would still have to deal with the outcomes of who their parents were when they were younger. In other words, the important "parent" to confront is the internalized person, not the living relative.

A similar appreciation for the irreversibility of the past applies, with special poignancy, to people whose backgrounds contain what they see as their own mistakes and transgressions. In my clinical experience, the most moving instances of the importance of substituting grief and regret for magical wishes to transform the past and its consequences involve parents who reared their children before they underwent personal therapy. The anguish of these people, who brought up their kids with the best of intentions but in the absence of understanding better ways to treat children at that time in their lives, can be excruciating to witness. Similarly, I have worked with people who felt extreme remorse about an abortion, an act of seemingly gratuitous cruelty, or a sin of omission such as inattention to the depression of someone they loved who then committed suicide. They cannot be glibly reassured, but they are deeply helped by having a place to grieve and be understood.

SUMMARY

I have tried to discuss in this chapter the features of individual human psychology that are often glossed over in therapists' training in case formulation because they are not so much "psychological" as part of the soil in which the client's psychology has taken root. Among those aspects of a person's psychology that a therapist must respect as "givens" are his or her temperament; congenital conditions; irreversible effects of physical trauma, illness, or addiction; unchangeable physical realities; unchangeable life circumstances; and personal history. Even though those features of someone's situation that are fixed and unchangeable are by definition not "dynamic," they have significant effects on an individual's psychodynamics and responsiveness to psychotherapy.

The main therapeutic implication of any facets of one's life that do not admit of change is the substitution of mourning and adaptation for self-hatred and magical wishes for transformation. I have stressed throughout this chapter the importance of the therapist's being straightforward and matter-of-fact when addressing areas about which the patient may feel shame, demoralization, and despair. I have also commented in numerous contexts about the therapist's inevitable resistances to helping clients face the implications of the unchangeable, in the hope that discussing such natural inhibitions will give practitioners the courage they need to jump in and name with their patients the nameless sorrows that have weighed down their lives.

CHAPTER FOUR

Assessing Developmental Issues

IN pursuing the preliminary and tentative understanding of a person that comprises a case formulation, most therapists put special emphasis on evaluating the developmental information gained in a clinical interview. Usually, in the client's individual history, there is a plausible answer to the focal diagnostic question, "Why is this person coming for help *now*?" If one can articulate the nature of the *person* (temperamentally and in terms of other fixed attributes), the nature of the current *stressors,* and nature of the *developmental issue* that those stressors activate for that person, one has the main outlines of a good dynamic formulation.

Many of the questions that therapists find useful to ask prospective clients are about maturation. In fact, the whole enterprise of taking a history assumes the developmental basis of psychopathology. For example, we commonly begin an intake session by asking why the person came for professional help at this particular time, and whether there have been previous times when similar problems arose. We inquire about what the person knows about his or her infancy and early childhood. We may ask for the person's earliest memory and for family stories about him or her. (Alfred Adler, 1931, observed that the first memory contained the major themes of an individual's personality. I know of many first memories that seem to confirm this, though I am not aware of research in this area. Many therapists have followed Adler on this point because their experience also attests to the richness of this line of inquiry.) We want to know about reactions to childhood separations, such as for day care or nursery school or elementary school, and about major moves or disruptions in the family and how the client reacted to them. We ask about childhood illnesses and accidents, about school history and work history, about the first sexual experience, sexual history, and current sexual life. By the time we have answers to these questions, we have a great deal to go on.

Because most analytic practitioners view psychotherapy as essentially an effort to rework previously thwarted processes of development (cf. Emde, 1990), a good understanding of normal development is essential. Some years ago, Gertrude and Rubin Blanck (Blanck & Blanck, 1974, 1979, 1986) gave the therapeutic community a comprehensive review of evolving psychoanalytic developmental theory, with the aim of helping therapists clarify what maturational tasks were unfinished or badly accomplished. Therapy can get people "back on track" if one knows what the track is. More recently, Greenspan (1997) has made a systematic integration of the newer discoveries in developmental psychology with psychotherapy theory. The excitement among analytic therapists about current research in infancy derives from the intimate connection they see between very early processes and clinical phenomena (see Sander, 1980; Lichtenberg, 1983, 1989; Stern, 1985; Dowling & Rothstein, 1989; Zeanah, Anders, Seifer, & Stern, 1989; Pine, 1990; Slade, 1996; Moskowitz, Monk, Kaye, & Ellman, 1997; Morgan, 1997; Silverman, 1998).

SOME CAUTIONARY AND ORIENTING COMMENTS ON PSYCHOANALYTIC DEVELOPMENTAL THEORY

From its inception, probably because of the profound influence that Darwin's thinking had on Freud, psychoanalytic theory has been epigenetic. In other words, it assumes that there is a naturally unfolding sequence of maturational changes in any organism that determines how it receives, interprets, and then shapes external influences. In Darwinian terms, a cataclysm like a flood will affect different species divergently, depending on their respective prior evolutionary histories and their unique adaptive capacities. Correspondingly, the same "objective" event in an individual's life will have radically contrasting implications for his or her psychology, depending on the developmental stage at which it makes its impact. The death of a parent for a child of two has dramatically different meanings and effects than if the child were four or nine or fifteen.

Consonant with the Piagetian concepts of assimilation and accommodation (Piaget, 1937; Wolff, 1970), analytic developmental theory assumes that the maturational stage of the individual both determines that person's experience of a given stressor and constructs the template for his or her interpreting the meaning and implications of future stressors. In adulthood, depending on what maturational issues have been more and less well worked out, specific stresses affect people in very different ways because they have radically different unconscious meanings. Thus, it is not possible to specify either the "obvious" independent effect of a particular stressor or the stimulus-independent description of a given time of life. External influence and developmental phase must be understood in combination, through identification with the sensorium of a unique human being.

Under stress, people tend to revert to the methods of coping that characterized an earlier developmental challenge that felt similar to their current situation: They "regress" to a point of "fixation." There is a more or less tacit assumption in psychoanalytic theory that the earlier a person has been faced with neglect or abuse or other overwhelming experience, the more vulnerable he or she is, and the more catastrophic and eventually cumulative are the effects of the traumatic circumstances. One of Freud's favorite metaphors (T. Reik, personal communication, January 29, 1969) for the interaction of maturation and stress was the image of an advancing army: As an army pursues its objectives, it is energized by victories and weakened by defeats. The earlier it undergoes defeat, the more incapacitated it is to meet future challenges. Early loss is not just a rout in one skirmish but sets the stage for losing subsequent battles as well.

This kind of thinking invited the conclusion that the most devastating psychopathologies, notably bipolar illness and the schizophrenic conditions, must reflect a psychological fixation on the oral level, resulting from defeats in mastering the expectable conflicts of that phase, while the less severe pathologies have their origins in problems from the oedipal phase or later. Although some scholars (e.g., Wilson, 1995) have challenged the facile assumption of "the earlier the worse," it remains a common supposition among analysts. Sass (1992, p. 21) argues that this assumption betrays an uncritical image of a "Great Chain of Being," a concept he has critiqued trenchantly for its misapplication to the phenomenological understanding of schizophrenia.

Interestingly, despite the "advancing army" metaphor and similar arguments, Freud did not consistently argue that early fixation produced the greatest problems; he repeatedly construed the oedipal phase as more consequential than preoedipal experience. While there is some empirical support for the general belief that more drastic pathologies reflect a fixation on earlier developmental stages (e.g., Silverman, Lachmann, & Milich, 1982), this assumption predates research on genetic contributants to the severer psychopathologies and can be misleading on at least two other counts: It underestimates the resilience of at least some infants, and it overestimates the resilience of older children and adults.

Research on infants (e.g., Tronick, Als, & Brazelton, 1977; Trevarthan, 1980; Fraiberg, 1980; Lichtenberg, 1983; Stern, 1985; Greenspan, 1989; Tyson & Tyson, 1990; Emde, 1991) has documented much more proactive, adaptive problem solving in the first months of life than we ever knew could be possible for young babies. Some children with constitutional advantages and empathic responsiveness can compensate remarkably for early deprivation and trauma. Ever since the pioneering work of Fraiberg and her colleagues (Fraiberg, 1980), clinical reports of successful early interventions with even seriously impaired infants of less than a year old have proliferated.

As for older individuals, as Bettelheim (1960) first noted, the people who survived the Nazi concentration camps best were not the ones that psychoanalysts would have endorsed as the healthiest. The experience of victimization was profoundly and permanently damaging to many people who seemed to have had a solid mastery of early conflicts. Trauma can override just about any developmental achievement (Herman, 1992). Less catastrophically, Wallerstein and Blakeslee (1989) have noted how even emotionally robust adults with good early parenting can be devastated by divorce. Although their research design had some weaknesses, and although there are great individual differences in reacting to divorce, most therapists have seen many clients who confirm what these writers describe. A difficult breakup can illuminate just how vulnerable are very competent and previously asymptomatic adults. Separation is a particularly painful kind of stress, and separation in a public and potentially humiliating context can undermine the psychological health of almost anyone.

Wolff (1996) contends that analytic developmental theory understands infants through adult constructs deduced in treatment, then, in circular fashion, uses the derived infantile concepts to interpret adults. Controversy about the relevance of infant research to clinical practice is currently a hot topic among analysts, one not easily represented fairly in a survey chapter such as this one. Still, the commonsensical idea that frustrations, disruptions, neglect, and mistreatment in the earliest phases of life have more far-reaching effects ultimately than those occurring later can be a useful orienting assumption if not applied uncritically. There are better grounds for reasoning forward from known infantile stressors than for reasoning backward to presumed causes. Thus, the fact that a man's mother was in a severe postpartum depression for most of the first year of his life should appropriately prompt an interviewer to ask him about first-year issues such as trust, capacity to soothe himself, capacity to regulate affect, and possible conflicts about closeness. But the information that a man has a problem with trust, self-soothing, affect regulation, and closeness should not automatically evoke the conclusion that his early mothering was faulty. Such leaps foreclose real understanding, substituting a derived model for important information.

My clinical experience has often supported Silvan Tomkins's (e.g., 1991) observation that stress in adulthood can activate early issues even when these were reasonably mastered in infancy. One should not jump from the observation of preoedipal themes to the conclusion that a person is somehow deeply, characterologically primitive. One can have significant issues involving orality, for example, despite having accomplished all the important tasks of the oedipal phase. Some light can perhaps be shed on the problem of applying developmental ideas to psychopathology by discriminating between the kinds of problems that seem to reflect an unconscious conflict and the kinds that seem to express a developmental arrest.

Assessing Whether a Problem Represents a Conflict or a Developmental Arrest

At the heart of Freud's model of the development of neurotic symptoms was the notion of unconscious conflict. As a prototype of this kind of symptom formation, let us consider the case of a fictitious Victorian woman I will call Amy, who has been brought up to believe that nice girls have no sexual desires. As she moves into late adolescence without any physical outlet for her sexual longing, she is tempted to masturbate. But because masturbation is looked upon as a depravity by her family and subculture, she cannot allow herself to let this idea into consciousness; it would create too much shame. Instead, she develops a hysterical glove paralysis. Her right hand, the one with which she would naturally masturbate if it were a practice she could accept, becomes useless. ("Glove paralysis" refers to anesthesia and immobility of the hand only, a classic conversion symptom not frequently seen in our era and culture but about as common in Freud's time as bulimia is in ours. This disability is prima facie hysterical in origin, because it is impossible to have a neurologically based paralysis of the hand without the arm being implicated.)

Freud would observe that the primary gain of the symptom is the removal of masturbation as a possibility, hence resolving the conflict, and that its "secondary gain" is that Amy may receive a certain amount of TLC that might partially meet the emotional needs that sexual gratification would more satisfactorily address. Therapy would require making Amy aware of the conflict, so that she could tolerate in herself the wish to enjoy her sexuality. She could still decide whether or not to masturbate; the point to the therapy would be to expand her autonomy and move into the area of personal choice something that had been automatically consigned to unconsciousness and suffused with shame and guilt.

Or consider an obsessive–compulsive symptom. The hypothetical Freudian patient Herman, a middle-aged accountant, cannot get through his day without carrying out numerous elaborate rituals involving turning off his stove and locking his door. He ruminates anxiously about what would happen if there were a gas leak (the house would blow up) or an intruder (its occupants could be killed). He has been bothered with these obsessive thoughts and compulsive rituals ever since he and his wife took into their home his ailing and cranky father. Conscious only of his filial love and duty toward the old man, he cares for him conscientiously, but he is rapidly becoming so immersed in his obsessions and compulsions that they interfere with the time he could be spending at his father's bedside or in other pursuits. Freud would say that the primary gain of Herman's symptom would be to handle the conflict between his conscious love for his father and his unconscious hatred and wish that the man would die. He would understand his fears of his father's being blown up or killed by an intruder as expressing an unacceptable, disavowed wish. The secondary gain of Herman's preoccupations is that they relieve him from some of the duties he would perform in the sickroom if he were free of obsession and compulsion. Therapy would involve making Herman conscious of the negative thoughts and feelings about his father so that he could choose in full awareness how much effort to put into his care.

This is elementary stuff, and even Freud's most straightforward cases were rarely this simple. I bring up these vignettes to illustrate the difference between etiologies of unconscious conflict and those expressing a developmental arrest. For both Herman and Amy, things had been going along well until a particular circumstance threw them psychologically off balance. For Amy, it was the press of adolescent hormones that upset her prior homeostasis. For Herman, it was the impingement of his sick father on his comfortable routines. Neither one could tolerate knowing some aspects of what they unconsciously felt about their respective situations. Both became symptomatic rather than face the shame or guilt of acknowledging sexual and aggressive drives that were culturally taboo. Their respective neuroses arose from the need to keep from consciousness the feelings of longing and resentment that their circumstances naturally provoked.

Suppose, however, that Amy's glove paralysis were only one symptom in a long series of hysterical afflictions; that these had gotten worse with adolescence, but that basically ever since she was a young child, she was vulnerable to fainting, vague indispositions, disturbances of sensation, and anesthesias not explainable physiologically; that in an initial interview, her therapist learned that she had always had a poor relationship with her mother, and that the idea of growing up to be like her had always filled Amy with horror. Then the explanation for her glove paralysis would be different and more complex, and the therapy required to address it would have to take into account that her current suffering was part of a much larger pattern of compromised development, during which Amy had never really been "well."

Let us suppose correspondingly that Herman had suffered from obsessions and compulsions all his life, and that the only reason he was coming to treatment now was that his wife was threatening to leave him because his ruminating and ritualizing were leaving her with the burden of care for both him and his ailing father; that his earliest memory was of his father's unrelenting criticism and his desperate efforts to be a good enough boy to earn the man's affection; that he had bathroom rituals, hand-washing rituals, stereotyped sexual practices, inhibited social relationships, and chronic superstitious behaviors. Again, this kind of clinical picture could not easily be reduced to a simple conflict, despite the fact that in some ways Herman's whole personality seems a study in conflict. And treatment would have to consist of a lot more than making unconscious fantasies conscious. For one thing, it would have to aim at establishing in the therapy, over a period of considerable time, a relationship that Herman could experience as noncritical.

These second hypothetical situations would inspire the inference by an interviewer that in each instance something had gone seriously wrong developmentally. The second version of Amy could not, for whatever reason, experience her mother as admirable enough to want to become like her in any respect. An interviewer might conclude that she had a profound fear of growing up, not just a culturally conditioned aversion to sexual enjoyment. The second Herman had never been able psychologically to separate and individuate from a father he still wanted so fervently to please. Both of them are maturationally stuck. They have failed to move reasonably adaptively through life because they are still trying to solve problems of its earliest years. Whereas in the first versions of their psychological circumstances they had matured satisfactorily and then regressed under stress, in the second version they never got beyond an infantile preoccupation that was badly addressed from infancy on. Their specific symptoms are the same in each scenario, but the meanings and implications of them are quite different.

Psychoanalytic literature in the second half of this century became very concerned with discriminating between these two types of presentation. Anna Freud, for example, wrote in 1970:

> In our times, the analyst's therapeutic ambition goes beyond the realm of conflict and the improvement of inadequate conflict solutions. It now embraces the basic faults, failures, defects, and deprivations, e.g., the whole range of adverse external and internal factors, and it aims at the correction of their consequences. Personally, I cannot help feeling that there are significant differences between the two therapeutic tasks and that every discussion of technique will need to take account of these. (p. 203)

The "basic faults" she mentions refer to the work of Michael Balint (e.g., 1968), one of the first analysts to explore issues such as core self-esteem as opposed to those of conflict between drive and inhibition. The work of Stolorow and Lachmann (1980) on distinguishing between defensive processes and a more pervasive maturational arrest they called "developmental prestages of defense" is another seminal paper on this kind of distinction. In the self psychology tradition, there is emphasis on two coexisting lines of development, one involving the drives and their objects, and the other involving the self and its felt wholeness, goodness, and consistency, a much more diffuse, developmentally implicated area. Kohut (1971, 1977) and his followers have consistently argued that analysts need to understand the latter processes better than Freud and most of his early successors did.

I am elaborating on this issue because it is critical to establishing a good case formulation. Every interviewer needs to try to understand with every patient how much of his or her suffering results from some immediate stimulus to unconscious, conflicted material, and how much of it reflects a kind of arrested psychological development. We also must keep in mind that maturation can be markedly uneven; that a person can have extraordinarily well-developed capabilities yet suffer from a crippling deficit in the area of, say, sexuality or the ability to be alone or the capacity to mourn, or comfort with competitiveness. "Fixation" is not a simple, unidimensional thing.

CLASSICAL AND POST-FREUDIAN DEVELOPMENTAL MODELS AND THEIR CLINICAL APPLICATIONS

In the rest of this chapter, I speak first from the vantage point of appreciating the permanent effects of early unfinished business, then from the perspective of understanding how certain kinds of stress can evoke maturational vulnerabilities in anyone, regardless of the success of his or her early development. In both sections, I follow mainstream psychoanalytic practice in emphasizing the first three Freudian stages of psychological development as most formative and of greatest importance in developing a narrative about a patient's individuality. Finally, I acquaint the reader with the literature on attachment style and its possible clinical implications.

First, a few paragraphs on psychoanalytic stage theory. Readers who are already familiar with this territory may want to skip over it. In this section, I oversimplify Freudian and post-Freudian theory for didactic purposes, omitting many interesting problems and complications in it. Because of the relevance of the overall model to the conceptualization of individual psychologies, I have written in a tone that presumes the usefulness of the basic Freudian outline even if one disagrees with aspects of it or finds some of its assumptions troubling. I should note that the tendency of analytic therapists to talk in Freudian developmental language does not indicate their agreement with him in such areas as whether to consider drive the main component of motivation, or pleasure the main aim of infant activity (see Silverman, 1998).

Freud's original theory of development stressed three "infantile" (i.e., preschool) stages, the oral, anal, and oedipal, each of which had predictable issues and conflicts, mastered differently depending on both the child's constitution and the caretakers' interventions. These were typically resolved by about age six into the main outlines of someone's permanent personality structure. (Freud also talked about minor transitional phases in the infantile era that applied differentially to the two sexes, including a urethral phase, a phallic phase, and a reverse or "negative" oedipal phase, but these have been less emphasized in the literature and include too many idiosyncratic issues to go into here.)

According to Freud, in the *oral* phase, the child's sensory experience is organized around the mouth, the chief organ for expression, exploration, and enjoyment, and the means of connection with the nursing mother from whom the child is not yet psychologically differentiated. From about eighteen months to three years, the child's preoccupation shifts to *anal* concerns, partly because of the maturation of the anal sphincter muscle and partly because the toilet training scenario typically represents the first conflict between the child's natural proclivities and the demands of civilization, represented by the child's caretakers. Associated infantile concerns involve struggles between compliance and rebellion, cleanliness and mess, giving and withholding, promptness and lateness, autonomy and shame, sadism and masochism—all very dyadic issues, in contrast to the more interconnected aura of the first year and a half. The dramas of this phase all seem to involve the question of agency. Colloquially, the Freudian "anal" phase has been nicknamed the "terrible twos" because of the intense pitting of the toddler's will against that of the parents at this time.

With the inception of the *oedipal* phase at about age three, the child has become cognitively capable of understanding that two other people can have a relationship in which he or she is not a player. The child's preoccupations shift to a fascination with issues about power, relationship, and identity. He or she gets very interested in sex differences, generating imagery about castration, mutilation, and other infantile theories about the distinctions between males and females. (Post-Freudian analytic researchers, starting with Galenson & Roiphe, 1974, have found that children are interested in this question much earlier than Freud believed. Nonetheless, youngsters do bring that prior interest into their experience of oedipal triangles with great intensity.) Children this age are raptly curious about the origins of babies, and they construct elaborate fantasies and experience associated jealousies about the parents' sexual life.

By somewhere around age three or four, normally developing children also have an awareness of personal agency that is not defined by dyadic power struggles as in the previous phase. They also come to an awareness of the reality of death, which, because of their unfinished sense of the independence of idea from action, makes them frightened by their natural wishes to get one parent out of the way and possess the other. Guilt and projected guilt, as in bedtime anxieties about hidden attackers, are typical. Fears of retribution for hostile wishes are eventually resolved by identification with primary caregivers, especially the parent with whom the child feels most competitive ("I can be like Daddy and have someone like Mommy when I grow up"). Children at this age need to idealize their caregivers, who, as self psychologists have noted (e.g., Kohut, 1977), must be attuned enough to be idealized in the first place and nondefensive enough to tolerate the child's deidealization. This normal, expectable dethroning of the parents starts around the end of the oedipal phase (when the kindergarten teacher starts knowing more than Mommy). A cardinal achievement of this developmental era is the attainment of a complex and well-internalized sense of conscience that is the natural consequence of complex identifications with childhood authorities. In analytic lingo, a mature superego replaces the primitive all-good and all-bad images of the previous stage.

Freud postulated a *latency* phase after age six or so, in which the child, because of having developed mature defenses, notably repression, that keep disturbing ideas out of consciousness, is temporarily relieved of the intensity of coping with powerful primal urges and can concentrate on learning and socialization. The hormonal assault of puberty ushers in *adolescence* and the final and sometimes stormy consolidation of all the early challenges and resolutions. With sexual maturity, it becomes possible for people to compress all their oral, anal, and oedipal issues into a pleasurable experience of adult *genitality,* an ideal condition characterized by a person's capacity to integrate love, aggression, dependency, and sexuality into a relationship with another person. Most of Freud's clinical writing emphasized the first three phases, as I have in this account, as he believed that neurotic problems in adulthood derive from universal "childhood neuroses."

Since Freud's time, psychoanalytic developmental theory has gone simultaneously in two opposite directions: (1) the dissection of the preoedipal stages into component subphases (e.g., in the work of Klein, 1946; Balint, 1960; Winnicott, 1965; Mahler, 1968; Mahler, Pine, & Bergman, 1975; the Blancks [G. Blanck & R. Blanck, 1974, 1979; R. Blanck & G. Blanck, 1986]; and Greenspan, 1989, 1997), and (2) the extension of the stage concept into later parts of the life cycle (e.g., the work of Erikson, 1950; Sullivan, 1953; Blos, 1962; Levinson, Darrow, Klein, Levinson, & McKee, 1978; Kaplan, 1984; and Osofsky & Diamond, 1988). These elaborations in both directions are important because of their implications for clinical intervention.

In addition, several theorists, Erikson being the most influential, have reinterpreted the classical prelatency stages, highlighting different developmental themes from the ones that were of central salience to Freud. In short, Erikson articulated the interpersonal tasks of the first three phases as opposed to the strivings for drive satisfaction that Freud had emphasized. He regarded his contribution as an elaboration of Freudian theory rather than a replacement of it. Most contemporary analysts follow Erikson in deemphasizing drive per se and in focusing on the quality of relatedness that characterizes each phase. Even those who follow Freud in stressing the organizing role of biological drives (e.g., Kernberg, 1992; Bernstein, 1993) emphasize their relational and affective implications more than Freud explicitly did.

In an intake interview, one needs to be sensitive to both infantile-through-preadolescent dilemmas, stages, and "moments" (Pine, 1985), and postpubertal crises, phases, and transitions. In assessing the psychology of any individual client, one must appreciate not only the nature of the person's current developmental challenges but also the nature of the earlier tasks to which they hearken back. For example, when working with a young adult, one needs to be aware of both the developmental tasks of the mid-twenties (most centrally, the attainment of deep intimacy with another person) and the early trust-versus-distrust issues that these maturational challenges restimulate. In passing, I should note that psychoanalytic knowledge of the latest phases of life is not well developed. Erikson frequently commented in his last decade that if he were writing his lifespan theory again, he would not have lumped everything from the sixties on into one category (see Erikson, 1997). Only by reaching old age himself did he emotionally appreciate the profound difference between the psychology of someone sixty-five and that of someone eighty-five. The integration of psychoanalytic ideas and gerontology has been underway for some time (e.g., Myers, 1984), but this book will doubtless reflect the limitations of the field as it now stands.

Developmental Aspects of Character Organization

A central diagnostic task of a clinical interview is assessing the developmental level at which a person is characterologically organized. Are the main issues with which the person repeatedly struggles those of the earliest phase of life, the one Freud called oral and Mahler called symbiotic? If so, the interviewer will hear themes such as the Eriksonian conflict between basic trust and distrust, the Sullivanian confusion of "me versus not me," R. D. Laing's (1965) "ontological insecurity," and other derivatives of the infant's struggle to define a sense of existence and personhood. The client will seem confused about what thoughts and feelings are inside him or her versus what is coming from outside. Reality testing will be problematic. Affect regulation may be difficult. One will have a hard time getting a picture of the main people in the client's world, as they will be described in vague or global ways that make them seem more like shadowy concepts than living beings. The patient may express uncertainty about his or her basic nature, including whether he or she is male or female, straight or gay, omnipotent or impotent, good or evil. The interviewer tends to feel overwhelmed in a vague and disturbing way.

Or is the person preoccupied with the themes and conflicts of the phase Freud called anal and Mahler called separation–individuation? If so, the clinician will feel a sense of dyadic struggle, of Erikson's (1950) "autonomy versus shame and doubt," of Sullivan's (1947) "good me versus bad me," of Mahler's (1971) "coming closer and darting away," of Masterson's (1976) engulfment versus abandonment depression, of Kernberg's (1975) alternating ego states. The *existence* of the self will not seem fragile, but the struggle between infantile helplessness and aggressive empowerment will be intense, and will induce in the interviewer very strong countertransference reactions (hostility, demoralization, and rescue fantasies are common). The images that the interviewer will derive of the people in the client's life will be stark and unnuanced; they will tend to appear as all-good and all-bad actors on the person's subjective stage. There may be evidence that the major players change frequently but always inhabit these all-good and all-bad roles. Reality testing will be adequate, but identity will seem tenuous, and primitive defenses such as denial, splitting, and projective identification will predominate in the person's efforts to solve problems.

Or does the person see the world through the lens of the oedipal phase? If so, one notes the client's susceptibility to conflicts about sexuality, aggression, and/or dependency in the context of an overall capacity for object constancy, an appreciation of the complexity of self and others, a tolerance for ambivalence, an ability to take an observing position toward his or her affective life, and a capacity to feel remorse and a sense of responsibility. Reality testing will be secure. The person's relationships will others will be marked by devotion, consideration, and the appreciation of the complexity of others. When speaking of the main people in his or her life, the patient will bring them alive as three-dimensional human beings in the diagnostician's mind. The oedipally organized individual comes across as a separate person with a strong sense of I-ness, and his or her suffering seems well demarcated into a particular area. The interviewer's countertransference tends to be benign.

This aspect of diagnosis is usually described as the assessment of whether one's client is organized characterologically at the symbiotic–psychotic, borderline, or neurotic level (we all have aspects of all of these, but usually one predominates). I have written in much more detail about the history and clinical implications of this aspect of conceptualization in *Psychoanalytic Diagnosis* (1994), where I also give an overview of the applicability of (1) supportive therapy, (2) expressive therapy, and (3) uncovering therapy, respectively, for the treatment of patients with these different kinds of character structures. I will give just one example here of how this aspect of the interviewer's formulation might eventually affect how the client is treated.

Supportive, expressive, and uncovering psychotherapies are all psychoanalytic, but they differ markedly. For example, a woman may be describing how upset she is that her boss has been critical. In supportive therapy, the clinician might say,

> "I can understand how disturbing that can be. You must find it hard to feel so angry and hurt. I hope you can manage to contain your feelings on the job so that your boss won't become any more critical."

In expressive therapy, an appropriate intervention might be,

> "You get very angry with me when you feel I don't appreciate how bad things are at work. When I sympathize with you about your job, you attack me for being impotent to change things there, yet when I suggest ways you might try to make things better, you get enraged because you feel I'm criticizing you. I think the feeling it creates in me, that nothing I do is right, is a feeling you struggle with all the time."

And in uncovering therapy, the clinician might simply ask,

> "Does your boss remind you of anyone?"

These are big differences in technique, and the choice to speak in the voice of one or the other depends mainly on a developmental assessment of an individual's personality organization.

Developmental Contributants to the Experience of Anxiety and Depression

An appreciation of different maturational aspects of personality structure is enormously helpful in evaluating the nature of a person's experience of anxiety or depression. When we listen to a patient who is anxious, we all tend to project into our understanding of that anxiety the kinds of issues that define our own anxious proclivities. But anxieties differ markedly, depending on whether their origin is in the symbiotic phase, the separation–individuation phase, or the oedipal phase. The first kind, generally referred to as *annihilation anxiety* (Hurvich, 1989), is the terror that the self will be overwhelmed, will be engulfed by another, will cease to exist. It is the kind of anxiety that an unmedicated person in an acute schizophrenic state emanates, and it is unbearable to witness, much less to feel. Most of us have powerful defenses against experiencing this kind of archaic dread in its intense infantile form and have trouble appreciating the depth of the pain of those whose defenses have not successfully contained it. Annihilation anxiety survives in the psychology of most adults in residual fears of intimacy. One can easily find evidence of people's anxiety that closeness with another person will threaten their independent existence.

The second kind, *separation anxiety,* affects all of us to some degree, as separations inevitably stimulate unconscious memory traces of frightening infantile disconnections, but it is an especially intense and central part of the experience of people organized at a borderline level of development. Separation anxiety also threatens the self with the specter of dissolution, though of a less radical kind than in annihilation anxiety. In the absence of the person to whom one is attached, one feels empty or insubstantial. It can be strong enough to keep a person in life-threatening situations, as when a battered spouse can deal more easily with the pain of physical abuse than the terror of aloneness. It can impel astonishing regressions and seemingly inexplicable explosions of hostility, even to the point of catathymic homicide (see Meloy, 1992).

The third kind of anxiety, oedipal or *superego anxiety,* involves fears of punishment for unacceptable sexual, aggressive, or dependent strivings. There is no threat to the perception of reality and identity of the self, but one's feeling of personal good-enough-ness may be seriously compromised. Despite the fact that it originates after the child has consolidated a sense of self and reality, oedipal-level anxiety can be quite intense, given that oedipal fantasies typically involve ideas of death and retribution. The experience of personal success is a common trigger for oedipal anxiety: If an achievement has for someone the emotional significance of victory over a parent, he or she may become very anxious or symptomatic in the unconscious expectation of punishment for that crime.

In *The Ego and the Mechanisms of Defense,* Anna Freud (1936) contrasted three kinds of anxiety, discriminated according to which psychic structure, the id, ego, or superego, had given rise to it. She called anxiety arising from the id "dread of the power of the instincts," emphasizing how the person suffering this anxiety felt in danger of being completely overwhelmed. She followed her father in labeling anxiety that originated in the ego as "signal anxiety"—a fear reaction signaling that something dangerous had happened previously when circumstances were like the ones the person is in now. Anxiety arising from the superego was simply called superego anxiety, and had the character of fear of punishment for unacceptable strivings.

Anna Freud was trying to explicate anxiety within the structural model her father had come to rather late in his career, a model that she and most analysts rightly regarded as a boon to clinical practice. Her work on this predated most psychoanalytic scholarship on infancy and the reformulation of Freud's developmental theory in the light of observations of young children. I regard her structural way of differentiating types of anxious reactions as compatible with psychoanalytic developmental ways one can do so. Dread of the power of the instincts is a natural concern of the earliest, symbiotic phase of development, when omnipotent fantasies prevail; signal anxiety arises once the child has separateness and the capacity to draw on memory; and superego anxiety reflects the achievements of the oedipal stage.

A therapist's understanding of how subjectively variable different anxiety states are makes clinical work much more effective than it would be if the treater regarded anxiety as a single, undifferentiated phenomenon. (Of course, this is how most advocates of pharmacological interventions construe it, not necessarily to the long-term benefit of the patient.) What kind of anxiety a person is suffering cannot be inferred automatically from his or her manifest situation. For example, if I come to a therapist in a state of mental anguish because I am having an illicit affair, there is no way the clinician can know initially whether I am overwhelmed by the power of the drives that have been activated by my falling in love with someone new, or whether I perceive unconsciously that it is dangerous to my safety, reputation, and family stability to have an affair, or whether I expect some internalized authority to punish me for committing adultery. If the therapist does not have a feel for the different kinds of anxious suffering and their different subjective meanings depending on which developmental issues have been stimulated, he or she is likely to project onto me whatever would be his or her own reaction to a similar situation—which may or may not fit my experience.

Similarly when someone is depressed, the sense of misery may be a psychotic-level sense that one's badness is so overwhelming as to render one unsalvageably and dangerously evil, or a borderline-level sense of despair, emptiness, and traumatic abandonment, or an neurotic-level conviction that it is hazardous to pursue happiness. A clinician's mode of providing comfort and hope to a depressed person depends to some extent on his or her having the right "take" on the subjective nature of the depression. Sympathy for anxious or depressive suffering is a natural reaction of compassionate people, but real empathy for the meaning of someone's suffering depends on an understanding of its particular nature and the developmental issues it represents.

Development, Life Stresses, and Psychopathology

People come for psychotherapy when something has happened in their lives that stimulates certain internal, often unconscious vulnerabilities. For one person the catalyst to seeking treatment is a personal rejection, for another a surprising success, for still another a sexual temptation, for yet another the demands of rearing a difficult child. Depending on the internal meanings of various stresses, it is not uncommon for someone to withstand gracefully what seem to observers to be major traumas, such as the deaths of several close relatives, and then to fall apart psychologically under the stress of what appears to other people to be a minor nuisance, such as an angry outburst from a competitive colleague.

A very frequent precipitant to seeking mental health services is an unconscious *anniversary reaction*—for example, the tenth year after a parent's death (the unconscious minds of people in our culture seem to go by the decimal system) or the client's reaching the age the parent had attained when he or she died. A related phenomenon from which one can infer an unconscious timekeeper is the depression that can hit a woman on the date when her aborted baby would have been expected to be born, or on the anniversaries of that date. Usually, people come to treatment unaware of these milestones, or have noted them and dismissed them as inconsequential.

Another common time for adults to seek therapy is the year that one of their children reaches the age at which they themselves had a traumatic experience. For example, if I was sexually molested at the age of seven, I am likely to become symptomatic in some way when my daughter reaches that age. If I lost my father at the age of thirteen, I would be at risk of psychopathology of some kind when my child becomes a teenager. This reaction seems to have several components, including (1) my unconscious reexperience of my own trauma, stimulated by my identification with my child; (2) a superstitious fear that she will go through the same thing I did and a wish to take that pain magically away from her and on to myself; (3) an unconscious envy and hostility toward her for *not* suffering as I did at her age, along with an indignation that she does not even feel grateful for her good luck or for the good mothering I am giving her that will protect her from going through what I did. It is important that interviewers look for these kinds of connections when trying to understand why someone has come for help *now*.

Some stressors have a natural tendency to activate the issues of a particular developmental phase. The experience of being arbitrarily oppressed or mentally played with and confused ("gaslighted" as per Calef & Weinshel, 1981) is likely to bring up the earliest questions about one's existence and sense of reality—that is, issues from the psychotic–symbiotic phase. The experience of losing a beloved person or being rejected by someone important will predictably stimulate the issues of the separation–individuation phase. The experience of sexual temptation or triangular competitive relationships will tend to bring up oedipal issues. It behooves us to understand this process so that we neither underpathologize nor overpathologize a patient on the basis of the developmental themes that have been catalyzed by a given stress. For example, a man who, after a disfiguring accident, finds himself feeling unreal, demoralized, and confused, cannot be assumed to have a symbiotic personality structure despite the fact that his feelings match the ones that express the problems of that stage of life. In his case, the nature of the stress he has gone through would induce those reactions in almost anyone.

Assessing Attachment Style

Development may proceed differently for people with different attachment styles, something we are still in the early stages of understanding.

It is important for clinicians not to equate a stable individual style of attachment with a developmental arrest. In the late 1970s, on the basis of a series of ingenious experiments inspired by Bowlby's (1969, 1973, 1980) work on attachment and separation, Mary Ainsworth and her colleagues (Ainsworth, Blehar, Waters, & Wall, 1978) delineated three distinct individual styles of attachment: *secure* (by far the largest category), *avoidant,* and *ambivalent–resistant.* All were seen as in the normal range of individual difference, except at the extreme ends of the avoidant and ambivalent continua.

Later research (Main & Solomon, 1986) established the existence of a fourth group, with a maladaptive style the researchers called *disorganized–disoriented* attachment. About eighty percent of maltreated infants (Osofsky, 1995) and forty to fifty percent of children with depressed or alcoholic mothers (Hertsgaard, 1995) fit this pattern. These children seek and then avoid attachment; show fear, sadness, confusion, aggression, panic, and apathy; have trouble concentrating; and often have dazed or trance-like facial expressions. The four patterns of attachment, which correlate with parents' attachment style (Main, Kaplan, & Cassidy, 1985), have been demonstrated to be stable at least through the school years (Kobak & Sceery, 1988). Clinical experience attests to the probability that these different ways of dealing with one's dependency are lifelong inclinations, but we await research to confirm this empirically. Meanwhile, many therapists have found an understanding of their patients' individual attachment styles to be critical to making therapeutic choices (see Stern, 1985, on some clinical implications of this body of infancy research).

SUMMARY

I have tried to give readers a brief exposure to psychoanalytic developmental theory, mentioning both its problems and limitations and its assets and clinical relevance. Psychoanalytic ideas about normal development are currently evolving very fast. Progress in empirical investigations of infancy and childhood, leading to the continuing refinement of attachment theory, cannot be fully represented in a chapter like this one despite its ongoing contribution to psychotherapy technique. I have touched, however, on the importance of assessing whether, in a given client, the psychopathology one is evaluating reflects a conflict or a developmental arrest. I have reviewed mainstream Freudian and post-

Freudian concepts of normal psychological maturation and discussed their implications for understanding both character structure and the meaning of different kinds of anxious and depressive affects. Finally, I have noted the role of particular stressors in shaping a person's individual psychological reaction.

CHAPTER FIVE

◖◖◗

Assessing Defense

AN appreciation of what has come to be known as "defensive" processes has characterized psychoanalytic thinking for a long time. Freud's original curiosity about psychopathology began with some observations (Freud, 1894) about what we would now consider the defense of dissociation or disavowal: How can somebody know and not know a thing at the same time? I covered the general topic of defense in Chapters Five and Six of *Psychoanalytic Diagnosis,* to which the reader is referred for conceptual background. For other summaries and viewpoints, one can also consult A. Freud (1936), Laughlin (1967), and Vaillant (1992). Here, my main concern is to illustrate how assessing a person's defensive tendencies contributes to making psychotherapy as effective as possible. I discuss both habitual defenses, those that have hardened into what Reich (1933) memorably called "character armor," and more reactive defenses that have been situationally provoked.

In a sense, the whole interview process stimulates defense, giving the clinician the opportunity to see how the patient copes with the stress of being invited to expose private and painful information to a stranger. People come to therapists with a potent combination of hope and shame. They want to reveal the psychological issues they are struggling with and, at the same time, they want to minimize them so that the therapist will not be as negative toward them as they themselves tend to be. They are simultaneously striving to be nondefensive and being propelled by their anxieties into being more defensive than usual. Most of the therapist's observations about defense will thus flow from the overall behavior of the person in the interview situation. Some of the specific questions that might highlight defensive functioning, however, include the following: What do you tend to do when you're anxious?

How do you comfort yourself when you're upset? Are there any favorite family stories about you that claim to capture your basic personality? What kinds of observations or criticisms or complaints do other people tend to make about you? How do you find yourself reacting to me?

Among analytic concepts, some of which are notoriously hard to study via empirical methods, defense has been one of the most carefully researched. Even though the essential nature of a defensive process is subjective and involuntary, and "defense" remains a hypothetical construct, there are ways of operationalizing processes such as "repression," "denial," "withdrawal," "idealization," and similar mechanisms that make them accessible to controlled experimentation. The concept of defense—sometimes under the nonpsychoanalytically tainted label of "coping style"—has even attained enough empirical validation to have been accepted into the DSM-IV (Axis VI: "Defensive Functioning Scale," under "Criteria Sets and Axes Provided for Further Study"), albeit as a kind of supplementary and optional category of diagnostic information. Vaillant and McCullough (1998) have recently presented research support for the diagnostic importance of defenses to Axis II descriptions, which in their current versions tend to emphasize observable behaviors more than internal motivations and thereby to sacrifice validity for reliability.

As Vaillant (1971) has pointed out, defenses can alter one's perception of any or all of the following: self, other, idea, or feeling. They can operate in the realm of cognition (e.g., rationalization, which seeks relief from painful states by manipulating ideas), emotion (e.g., reaction formation, which handles an upsetting feeling by turning it into its opposite), behavior (e.g., acting out, which provides escape from painful conflicts by external enactments), or some combination of these (e.g., reversal, which operates via cognition and behavior: "I'm not the one who feels X—*you* are, and so I will treat you in a way that relieves your presumed feeling").

Although there is general agreement among psychoanalytic scholars that some defenses constitute better overall adaptations than others (e.g., Laughlin, 1967; Kernberg, 1984), and although there is a solid empirical basis for assuming that defenses can be put into a hierarchy of relative psychopathology (Weinstock, 1967; Haan, 1977; Vaillant, 1977), there is no normative pattern of defense by reference to which the unhealthy deviate from the healthy. Among therapists, Kernberg's (e.g., 1984) rationale for distinguishing between primitive, or primary,

and secondary, or mature, defenses is probably the most widely accepted. Kernberg argues:

> Repression and such related high-level mechanisms as reaction formation, isolation, undoing, intellectualization, and rationalization protect the ego from intrapsychic conflicts by the rejection of a drive derivative or its ideational representation, or both, from the conscious ego. Splitting and other related mechanisms protect the ego from conflicts by means of dissociation or actively keeping apart contradictory experiences of the self and significant others. (p. 15)

The "other related mechanisms" include primitive idealization, projective identification, denial, omnipotence, and primitive devaluation. I have noted (McWilliams, 1994, p. 98) that the defenses we tend to consider more archaic involve the boundary between the self and the outer world, whereas those we consider higher-order processes deal with internal boundaries, such as those between the ego or superego and the id, or between the observing and experiencing parts of the ego.

People's defensive patterns are almost as individual as their voice or their fingerprints. Some people use sadness as a defense against anger, while others get angry to defend against sadness. Some defend against a pervasive underlying shame; others seek not to feel guilt. Some have an extensive repertoire of defenses, while others perseverate with one or two tried-and-true mechanisms, no matter what the circumstances. In order to help a person, we need to appreciate the particular way in which he or she is using thoughts, feelings, and actions to relieve upsetting internal states.

CLINICAL VERSUS RESEARCH CONSIDERATIONS IN ASSESSMENT OF DEFENSE

For research purposes, nosologies that emphasize observable behaviors are preferable to those that make use of internal and inferred processes. But for clinical purposes, it is more important to know the meaning of a person's behavior than to describe that behavior accurately the way an external observer would. The phenomenon of antisocial personality disorder or psychopathy, in the older language of descriptive psychiatry and psychoanalysis, nicely illustrates the limitations of assessment according to mostly observable behavior, assessment that ignores the significance of a person's inferred defensive proclivities. Since the 1980 edition, the DSM has relied heavily on the research of Lee Robins (e.g., 1966), a sociologist interested in antisocial behavior, because her definitions of psychopathic phenomena are descriptive rather than inferential, and empirically determined rather than theoretically derived. Her behavioral, observable criteria for assessing antisocial personality disorder (a term that itself reflects the sociologist's interest in phenomena that deviate from conventional norms, in contrast with the psychotherapist's concern with motivation and personal meaning) are thus highly adaptable to conventional research. Reflecting its dependence on Robins's work, the DSM-IV has seven criteria for Antisocial Personality Disorder, only one of which, "lack of remorse," is internal.

But to a therapist, the critical indicators of a psychopathic orientation are almost exclusively internal. They include consistently observed and well-documented phenomena such as emotional insincerity (Cleckley, 1941), defects of conscience (Johnson, 1949), contemptuous delight at "getting over on" others (Bursten, 1973), attraction to extreme stimulation (Hare, 1978), lack of empathy (Hare, 1991), egocentricity or grandiosity (Cleckley, 1941; Hare, 1991), obliviousness to affects (Modell, 1975) except perhaps for rage and envy (Meloy, 1988), and perhaps most centrally (and vital to the argument in this chapter), reliance on the primitive defense of omnipotent control (Kernberg, 1984; Meloy, 1988; Akhtar, 1992).

Therapists see many people who do not, at least on the basis of what can be observed in an initial interview, meet the DSM criteria for Antisocial Personality Disorder of engaging in unlawful behaviors (1), acting impulsively (3), displaying overt irritability and aggressiveness (4), showing reckless disregard for the safety of self and others (5), or behaving irresponsibly (6). Some people who take a chronically manipulative, unempathic, power-oriented approach to life are on the surface quite conventional, amiable folks. But experienced clinicians may sense the presence of psychopathy from evidence that a person relies chronically on the defense of omnipotent control. They may infer this from a woman's somewhat intrusive questions, from the charming way a man holds the door open for his female therapist, or from the glee with which a corporate executive describes his or her role in a hostile takeover. Many superficially appealing, apparently law-abiding middle-class people with none of the overt DSM criteria will reveal their antisocial side when given projective tests (Gacano & Meloy, 1994).

The DSM criteria lend themselves to overdiagnosis of psychopathy among people in marginal subgroups, such as adolescent gangs and

criminal organizations, and underdiagnosis of it among those who succeed in mainstream roles. They more readily categorize as having Antisocial Personality Disorder those people who are poor or unconnected
with powerful others, and who are therefore less likely to be bailed out
of the difficulties that their personalities create. It is hardly rare, however, to find psychopathic people in politics, in the business community,
the military, the entertainment industry—in any roles in which the opportunity to wield power is great. The DSM, in other words, can lead
one to identify *unsuccessful* psychopathic people rather easily (e.g.,
those who have been typed as conduct disordered in childhood or arrested for illegal acts in adolescence or adulthood) but provides little
help in identifying those whose capacity to con is highly developed and
effective.

Understanding the internal subjective world of the psychopathi-
cally inclined person is much more useful therapeutically than locating
him or her in an "antisocial" *role*. Clinical ramifications of such understanding include the importance of the therapist's taking an explicitly
power-oriented stance with the client, demonstrating incorruptibility,
and making interventions that assume a utilitarian rather than a moral
compass in decision making (Greenwald, 1958; Meloy, 1988, 1992;
Akhtar, 1992; McWilliams, 1994). In many cases, especially in subtler
ones in which a person's antisocial proclivities are not picked up by the
schools or the legal system, the therapist's assessment of defense will be
critical. That assessment can alert the interviewer to antisocial dynamics long before the behavioral consequences of a psychopathic psychology become evident—an outcome of special importance in the case of
this diagnosis. Psychopathic people often come to treatment in the service of a manipulation (e.g., with a view to the therapist's testifying on
their behalf or qualifying them for disability income, or colluding in the
fiction that because they have sought therapy, they are earnestly trying
to change some destructive pattern that they fear is about to be exposed).

Although a particularly compelling one, psychopathy is only one
exemplar of the importance of assessing the nature of a client's relatively invisible defense system. Just as a person's reliance on omnipotent
control in the interview situation alerts a therapist to a possible psychopathic streak in the interviewee, habitual reliance on another defense or
constellation of defenses has been associated with (or, in my way of
thinking, is definitional of) certain characterological tendencies. Each
tendency has a distinguished history of clinical and theoretical investigation. Reliance on splitting, projective identification, and other "prim-

itive" defenses is associated with borderline-level personality organization (Kernberg, 1975); idealization and devaluation suggest narcissism (Kohut, 1971; Kernberg, 1975; Bach, 1985); withdrawal into fantasy indicates schizoid tendencies (Guntrip, 1969); reaction formation and projective defenses constitute a paranoid process (Meissner, 1978; Karon, 1989); regression, conversion, and somatization indicate a psychosomatic vulnerability and associated alexithymia, the inability to put words to feelings (Sifneos, 1973; McDougall, 1989); introjection and turning against the self are implicated in depressive and masochistic psychologies (Menaker, 1953; Berliner, 1958; Laughlin, 1967); denial is the hallmark of mania (Akhtar, 1992); displacement and symbolization suggest phobic attitudes (MacKinnon & Michels, 1971; Nemiah, 1973); isolation of affect, rationalization, moralization, compartmentalization, and intellectualization are definitional of obsessional tendencies (Shapiro, 1965; Salzman, 1980); undoing is an essential defense in compulsivity (Freud, 1926); repression and sexualization imply hysterical issues (Shapiro, 1965; Horowitz, 1991); dissociative reactions characterize posttraumatic states of mind (Putnam, 1989; Kluft, 1991; Davies & Frawley, 1993). This way of thinking is of course subject to all the criticisms about labeling and pathologizing for which many have faulted the DSM and descriptive psychiatric diagnosis in general, but the labels associated with a sophisticated understanding of defense are at least larger, more complex constructs, attached to bodies of literature from which a conscientious clinician can derive extensive knowledge of how to orient treatment.

CHARACTEROLOGICAL VERSUS SITUATIONAL DEFENSIVE REACTIONS

A specific defensive reaction can be determined mostly by people's individual character structure or by the situation in which they find themselves, as was true with the maturational issues discussed in the previous chapter. As an example of a characterological defensive pattern, consider a man with a paranoid personality. The defining indicator of paranoid functioning is dependence on the defense of projection. A man who is characterologically paranoid will use projection in almost every circumstance. If he is cut off by a car, he will project his rage onto the driver, generating the conviction that the perpetrator had a hostile intent to impede him. If he feels a threatening sexual attraction to someone, he will attribute his erotic wishes to the other party, condemning that person for lustfulness. If he is with a person who provokes his envy, he may focus on an admirable quality in himself and attribute the envy to the other person. In therapy, he will project his personal preoccupations into his understanding of the therapist's communications, wondering whether the therapist's tired look means that she finds him boring, or whether the therapist's passing comment about the weather contained some hidden innuendo about his sexual orientation. He may be uncannily perceptive about emotions in others, including those of a therapist, yet wildly off base and self-referential in his interpretation of the *meaning* of any given feeling.

It can be difficult to differentiate a characterologically paranoid person from someone in a situation that by its nature tends to stimulate paranoia. Trauma, given its effect in shattering a person's prior expectations and basic security, creates paranoid aftereffects in previously nonparanoid people (Herman, 1992). Ambiguous situations also invite projection, as analytic therapists well know; with healthier clients, we deliberately convey only minimal information about ourselves in order to explore what they project on to us. In the absence of adequate external information, people will call upon internal data to understand what is happening to them. The more painful their circumstances, the more they need to try to comprehend them by reference to the only information they have: their inner state. Thus, any condition in which a person feels stirred up emotionally (e.g., when treated arbitrarily or unfairly), and in which he or she has inadequate information about what is going on, will elicit projection. When people feel ashamed, they frequently assume that someone is trying to shame them. When they feel hurt, they often ascribe the wish to hurt to the injurious party. They are only sometimes right, of course, since the effects of people's actions are often quite distinct from the motivations that give rise to them.

All defensive reactions constitute a blend of personal inclinations and situational provocations. It is clinically useful to assess whether any given reaction represents more the former or the latter. When a client reports a particularly dehumanizing work situation and announces that her boss is out to get her, the apparently paranoid quality of her conclusion may reflect mostly her character structure or mostly an adaptation to a reality that tends to induce projection. One clinical basis for determining whether a defense is more characterological or more situational is the therapist's inner subjective response to the patient. If the projective defense is predominantly characterological, the interviewer will be struck with how instantly and unreflectively the patient projects on to him or her. If it is mainly reactive, the therapist will feel taken in as separate, interesting, and potentially helpful despite the client's agitation about a problematic situation. Tactful questions about the person's background and behavior outside the disturbing arena will also help to clarify what is going on. In reactive paranoia, the projective responses will be confined to the situation that induces the reaction; for example, a person with reactive paranoia who feels persecuted at work will not report feeling persecuted by family members or close friends.

To illustrate the same point via a different defense, consider denial, another mechanism that can be automatically set off by overwhelming life events. The first response any of us tends to make when presented with terrible news is, "Oh, no!" Most of us are pretty good intuitively at knowing the difference between someone who is characterologically manic, and who therefore (by definition) uses denial in virtually every circumstance, and someone who is coping with a life challenge, such as a diagnosis of cancer, that has provoked some amount of denial until the person works out more adaptive ways of coping with the disaster. Again, the interviewer's assessment of whether a person is in a transient, situationally induced state of denial or whether he or she habitually denies all upsetting information depends on an attunement to the general tone of an interview. The usual countertransference to a characterologically manic or hypomanic person is a sense of things spinning, moving very fast, being confusing, being unintegrated with feelings. The rather common misdiagnosis of people in serious manic episodes or with hypomanic personalities as less disturbed than they in fact are probably reflects therapists' natural empathy for the uses of denial in many situations—so much so that the characterological basis for a cyclothymic person's problem may be overlooked.

CLINICAL IMPLICATIONS OF ASSESSING DEFENSE

Long-Term versus Short-Term Implications

The traditional rationale for making a careful assessment of a person's stable defensive organization is that in long-term analytic therapy, a pattern of defense can be altered in ways that free people up to have richer experiences and a broader range of options. Clients can learn to identify when they are about to go "on automatic" with a particular defensive strategy and pause to wonder whether that is the most effective response to a situation. They can substitute thoughtful, voluntary actions for unreflective, involuntary, and often self-defeating ones. They can move toward more mature versions of any particular defensive style (e.g., from complete isolation of affect to a somewhat intellectualized acknowledgment of the presence of feelings, or from primitive to mature idealization). They can master a wider and more effective repertoire of coping mechanisms.

In this era of economic pressures to do the minimum therapeutically, most people still appreciate intuitively that what they have come to therapy to work on will take a long time. Some of them are able and willing to make the investments that this kind of growth requires. There are also people—for example, those who depend automatically on radical and total kinds of dissociation—whose defenses are so maladaptive that even third-party payers are occasionally willing to concede that they need long-term treatment to change their defensive pattern. But even in other instances, when one can do only short-term work or crisis intervention, it is of great value to have an understanding of a person's characterological defenses. This knowledge allows us to choose a style of intervention that is most likely to be assimilated by a particular patient.

Let me begin with what most clinicians consider the ideal situation: The client is self-referred, motivated for treatment, able to afford it, and willing to stick with it as long as it takes to do significant work on the sources, not just the current manifestations, of recurrent psychological problems. Under these circumstances, if one determines that the defenses the patient is using to deal with a particular life stress are both maladaptive and situational, one can point them out and encourage the person to consider other ways of addressing the problem. For example, consider an otherwise emotionally involved man who is reacting to a parent's terminal illness with a general pattern of withdrawal. One can tell him that although it is natural for people to try to avoid painful situations, he may regret later that he was not closer to his father during the last months of his life. One can explore his fears that to spend time with his dying father will bring on a deep grief and wonder with him why it would be so terrible to feel the pain that naturally accompanies loss. One can explore whatever fantasies he has about what it would mean to "lose control" over his emotions. One can point out that his withdrawal is not magically extending his father's life or making his final days more bearable. One can brainstorm about other ways he could handle his grief that would be more proactive and ultimately satisfying to him and his family. And so forth.

If, on the other hand, one determines that a patient's current defenses are both maladaptive and characterological, the clinical challenge is significantly greater. In the prior example, in which a relatively expressive, connected man finds himself inexplicably withdrawing, the therapist can access the part of the patient that can see the withdrawal as aberrant and self-defeating. But if a person in the same situation had a lifelong pattern of responding to unpleasant realities by withdrawing, there would be no "observing" part of him to access. His tendency to withdraw would be so natural and automatic to him that he could not initially conceive of handling things another way. Like the air he breathes, his defensive pattern would feel so familiar to him that he could not even conceptualize it as something he could look at and think about.

In cases like these, where a given defense is so ingrained that it is invisible to the person using it, standard analytic practice has been to spend the first months and even years of therapy making ego-alien what has been ego-syntonic. Direct, early interpretation of the defense will be experienced not as helpful but as critical and undermining, because the person's basic *modus vivendi* is under attack and he or she cannot imagine operating any other way. The therapist must work patiently with such a client, only gradually raising questions about other possible ways to address the stresses he or she encounters. One cannot remove a defense when it is the main structure by which a person attempts to cope. There are numerous books in the psychoanalytic literature that address themselves entirely to this long-term therapeutic process as it applies to a particular kind of character. For example, Mueller and Aniskiewitz (1986) have written about how to work with hysterical patients, who use repression, regression, conversion, and acting out; Salzman (1980) has done it for obsessional clients, who use isolation, compartmentalization, rationalization, intellectualization, and undoing; Davies and Frawley (1993) have done it for people who habitually dissociate.

What about those instances where, for whatever reason, we can do only short-term work or crisis intervention? It is still of value to appreciate that a defense is characterological, even though it is no more confrontable in a situation of limited time than it is in the early phases of an open-ended, long-term contract. Consider a woman with a basically masochistic character structure—a shorthand way of saying that she depends habitually and automatically on the defenses of turning against the self and reversal. She is able to pursue her own needs only by projecting them on to others and taking care of those others; when it comes to care of herself, she is relentlessly self-effacing. In long-term therapy, one could reasonably expect such a person to integrate and better handle the drives and needs that are denied, projected, and addressed in other people. But in the short run, one must simply appreciate that this is the way this woman deals with aspects of herself that she has come to regard as unacceptable, and one must therefore work *within* that psychology. Thus, if one is trying to influence such a client to consider adopting different behavior toward a partner who is mistreating her, one cannot make a frontal assault on her defenses and announce, "He's being abusive! You shouldn't put up with that. Tell him if he doesn't stop, you'll be out of there!" (If this approach worked, there would be a lot fewer people in psychotherapy, for it seems to be the treatment of choice of most nonprofessionals trying to help their victimized acquaintances.)

Frontal attacks on defenses present the defended person with only two options: (1) Give up the defense and, in the absence of having developed coping mechanisms to substitute for it, become overwhelmed with anxiety, shame, or guilt; or (2) fight off the person who is assaulting one's cherished method for coping with life. People almost always choose the latter. Sometimes they can choose the former via an idealization of the therapist that compensates for the loss of their defense ("I will comply, based on my belief that my therapist is a person of enormous superiority to me. My anxieties about behaving out of character are compensated by my conviction that my therapist knows better than I do what is good for me"). But then one has only changed the locus of the problem: Now the therapist is the dominating one, giving orders with which the client complies at the price of his or her dignity and autonomy. A specific self-defeating behavior has been stopped, and the person's dependence has been shifted to a better object, but the client's disposition to defer has been reinforced rather than weakened.

Because direct assaults on favored defenses are thus doomed, most therapists in short-term situations learn ways to sidestep and finesse clients' defensive patterns, or to use their defenses in the service of their growth rather than their paralysis. With the hypothetical masochistic woman, one stands a far greater chance of persuading her to become more assertive if one can frame one's interventions in a language that is not too far from her defensive needs. For instance, one can say,

"I wonder if it's really good for Bob to be able to push you around like that. Don't you worry that it's corrupting for him to get away with being a bully? That's certainly not a self-image he can be proud of. Is there a way you could respond to his demands that would give him more of a sense of being a reasonable grown-up, negotiating conflicts from a position of equality?"

A woman who is compelled for unconscious reasons to evaluate her actions always from the view of what is good for others may be able to rethink habitual behaviors if she can see that they do not contribute to a healthy pattern for the other person.

To take a dramatically contrasting example of this principle of appreciating someone's defenses and framing one's comments in ways that avoid doing violence to that person's habitual ways of thinking, feeling, and behaving, consider the challenge of therapeutic interventions with characterologically psychopathic clients. A man with an antisocial personality will not be able to assimilate interpretations that fail to take his ubiquitous use of the defense of omnipotent control into account. Any experienced police officer knows that to get a perpetrator to cop to a crime, one cannot simply mount a charge against his need to see himself as a person who is always on top of things. Thus, statements such as "You got out of control," which offer an excuse, but one based on weakness, will not promote a confession. Nor will appeals to a sense of guilt (e.g., "You have to think about the effects on the victims"). Omnipotence does not admit of imperfection or moral fault; it is only about power. So instead of saying to a murderer, "For the sake of the victim's family, you need to admit what you've done," cops learn to say, "Gee, if you claim you weren't aware of what you were doing, people will think you're mentally disturbed. Is that how you want them to see you?" Most antisocial people would rather risk incarceration than be seen as weak and deranged.

The therapeutic analogue to this forensic example is the psychopathic client that the therapist wants to get to stop lying. Empathic reflections of why the person needs to deceive will not elicit honesty, since someone trying to feel omnipotent will not acknowledge need. Statements that implicitly moralize will be similarly fought off, disparaged as the hypocritical rationalizations of a person without enough sense to see how brutal life is. Instead, the therapist can say,

> "Look, you're good. You're very convincing, and I can see that even though I encourage you to come clean here, you still can't resist the temptation to lie to me. And I'm sure there will be plenty of times when you'll get over on me. But it's not really in your interest to do that here, since telling me fairy tales only wastes your money and

my time. You're the expert on your psychology: How can I get you
to find the guts to tell the truth here?"

By accepting the person's grandiose sense of himself and associating
truthfulness with courage, a power position, the therapist maximizes
the possibilities that the patient will cooperate.

Systematically Exposing versus "Going Under" Defenses

In circumstances where one has the time and the commitment from a
client to work in depth on personality issues, one still needs to assess
that person's particular defensive structure in order to know what style
of communication is most likely to reach him or her. The classical psychoanalytic approach to doing defense analysis is to go "from surface
to depth" (Fenichel, 1941), that is, to visualize the patient's mental organization as layered, with each layer defending against the content of a
deeper layer. The therapist systematically and tactfully addresses the
conscious or nearly conscious parts of the person's experience. As the
client feels increasingly known and safe, each underlying layer of defense or meaning or experience emerges, and the therapist deals with
each as it appears in the treatment relationship.

For example, a person with hysterical features often presents in an
ingratiating way. Beneath that surface presentation, one typically finds
distrust, hostility, and competition. Underneath these more truculent attitudes are serious fears and a profound sense of personal vulnerability.
In other words, the ingratiation is a defense against hostile attitudes,
which in turn defend against fear and a subjective sense of weakness. In
working with a hysterically organized person who manifested these dynamics, one would initially say something like, "I notice that you always agree with me and are very deferential in general. Surely, sometimes you don't feel quite that agreeable." Such a comment typically
provokes self-scrutiny by the patient, whose defensive system has been
challenged but not so much as to feel overly threatening. He or she
might then associate to having a general style of ingratiation, and the
therapist could then explore with the patient the question of what attitudes the ingratiation might be covering up.

If instead one tried to "go under" the defensive structure with an
interpretation such as, "I think you're really hostile toward me," or
"Perhaps underneath that facade of ingratiation you're scared to death
of me," most patients would either find that attribution too far from
their conscious experience to access any awareness of the ascribed feel-

ing, or would feel traumatically exposed and too threatened to cooperate further with the treatment. This is assuming that the interpretation is correct, which is, of course, assuming too much. In fact, one of the traditional reasons for going carefully from surface to depth is that one can be drastically off base when hypothesizing about the functions of various defenses, and one wants, whenever possible, to work at a level where a patient can take or leave what the therapist says, and do so with the confidence that comes from being in touch with the level of experience under discussion.

Another example of the appropriateness of interpreting from surface to depth would be the patient with obsessive–compulsive features whose clinical presentation is a highly intellectualized and cooperative demeanor that covers over an argumentative, nitpicking attitude that defends against a deep shame. The therapist would generally start addressing not the sense of shame but the person's penchant for intellectualization. An exploration of this would typically lead to the more aggressive components of the patient's personality. As the client felt increasingly understood and accepted despite the unpleasantness of such hostile attitudes, the hostility would eventually soften up and allow the areas of shame to emerge. If one tried to access the shame without going through the defenses against it, layer by layer, one would risk either mortifying the patient or having one's interpretation turned to ice by a penchant for intellectualizing.

Interpreting from surface to depth is almost always the approach of choice, and most therapists do this naturally and intuitively, whether or not they have been trained in psychoanalytic metapsychology. "Start where the patient is" and "Don't mess with a defense until the person has something to replace it with" are the kinds of things that experienced supervisors tell their students every day. But there are some kinds of defensive patterns that require more of a depth-charge strategy from the clinician. Specifically, both hypomanic and paranoid patients need therapists who understand the need to "go under" rather than to stay at the top of their personal hierarchy of defenses.

"Hypomanic" or "cyclothymic" are psychiatric labels for a personality pattern in which denial is the front-line defense. Hypomanic people are frequently "up" in terms of their mood and may have all the ebullience, charm, wit, and energy of the life of the party. Their histories attest, however, to profound difficulties with intimacy and genuineness, and they tend to bolt from relationships that start to feel important to them. They are subject to abrupt swings into depression whenever their defense of denial wears thin, exposing pain about loss, vulnerability, mortality, and other unpalatable facts of life that the rest of us are not quite so primitively defended against facing. They typically come to therapy to get help with depressive plunges and are famous for bolting from therapy as soon as their mood goes up again. Interviewers often react to them as charming and feel some surprise that such an engaging, lighthearted person can report periodic battles with profound despair.

Hypomanic people are virtuosos at denial. Because denial is such a rigid, all-or-nothing defense, it cannot be gently addressed in the surface-to-depth manner that works best with other clients. Anyone who has experience with substance abuse, a condition in which denial is notoriously involved, knows that one sometimes has to go after this defense with both barrels. The therapist who would never take on a person with an ingratiating defense by announcing, "You're trying to ingratiate yourself with me. Stop it!" might, especially under circumstances in which a client is behaving self-destructively, exclaim, "You're in denial. Get real!" Anything less assaultive than this—say, for instance, a tactful question along the lines of "Do you worry that your drinking might be getting out of control?"—typically elicits more denial.

With hypomanic patients, the characterological nature of their denial (as opposed to its operating in a specific area, like an addiction) requires therapists to find creative ways to address it without making the full-scale frontal attack that would only be self-defeating. Clinical experience suggests that going directly to depth—bypassing the surface and ignoring the layer of denial—is often the technique of choice. For example, a cyclothymic woman who is behaving in driven and self-destructive ways in the context of the therapist's upcoming vacation could be told, "You're probably not conscious of this, but I'm pretty convinced that you're reacting to my upcoming vacation with a lot of anxiety, based on some unconscious fears that I won't come back." Such an intervention may be accepted or rejected, but it will penetrate. If the therapist were instead to ask, in the surface-to-depth manner that makes sense for other kinds of patients, "I wonder if your recent spurt of drinking and picking up men has anything to do with my upcoming vacation," the client would most likely respond with denial and there would be no place to go.

Paranoid patients also require a bypassing of defense to go to what is defended against, but for somewhat different reasons. Paranoid people are terribly afraid at an unconscious level that they are dangerously powerful. Their use of rigid and primitive defenses such as denial, reaction formation, and projection to deal with this internal feeling of a threatening badness creates their sense that the threat will come from outside. For at least two reasons, they need the therapist to go under their defensive structure to the feelings and needs that invoke their defenses: (1) They need to see the therapist as tough and smart, because otherwise, they unconsciously fear that they will damage him or her with their evil power, and (2) they have done so many transformations of a simple feeling by the time they present what is manifestly on their minds that working from surface to depth will never get down to their basic concerns.

To illustrate the second point, consider the paranoid woman who expresses to the therapist a boiling outrage springing from the conviction that her husband is seeing another woman, something for which there seems to be no evidence. The therapist may be able to see that this preoccupation started with a simple feeling of loneliness and the wish to be close to a female friend. It then became transformed by several rigid defenses in succession, as follows:

> "Since I am bad, my need for love from a woman must reflect my depravity. The need feels so strong I experience it as erotic. That's unacceptable. Maybe she's the one putting these homosexual thoughts in my mind. She's the bad one, not me. And I'm not the one who desires her—it's my husband."

Thus, via denial, reaction formation, projection, and displacement, a simple need is transformed into a paranoid preoccupation. The therapist who tried to work from surface to depth ("What comes to mind about your idea that your husband is having an affair?") would elicit only more paranoid rumination.

But a therapist might be able to make contact with this woman by saying something like, "I think you've been feeling quite lonely lately, so naturally you're worried about the fidelity of those you depend on." This could lead to some problem-solving discussion about the normality of loneliness and the options the patient has to find friends. Another bypassing kind of intervention would be, "I have the strong sense that unconsciously you have this conviction that there is something terrible and dangerous about you. Maybe at some irrational level you feel your husband sees your badness and would naturally reject you for someone else." Again, a paranoid person would be likely to be interested in this concept, and both she and the therapist could get some relief from the relentlessness of the paranoid concerns that her defenses have created.

SUMMARY

In this chapter, I have made some orienting comments on the psychoanalytic concept of defense, emphasizing the importance to clinical practice of understanding the internal, subjective, and reflexive ways people try to protect themselves from suffering. I have tried to help the reader distinguish characterological defensive reactions from those provoked by particular stresses, and I have addressed some of the clinical implications of making that distinction. In instances where a person's defenses have crystallized to the extent that he or she can legitimately be seen as having a personality disorder, I have noted some technical implications of this observation for long-term and short-term treatments, respectively. Finally, I have mentioned the conditions under which the usual wisdom of working with defenses "from surface to depth" does not apply.

As Vaillant and McCullough have observed (1998, p. 154), we all display more mature dynamics when we feel understood. Understanding how a person defends against painful emotions is critical to understanding his or her general psychology. Learning how to convey that understanding in ways that those very defenses will not screen out or distort is essential to the art of psychotherapy.

CHAPTER SIX

《@

Assessing Affects

THE psychoanalytic tradition has had a complicated theoretical history, one in which clinical practice and the theory on which it is ostensibly based have not always been entirely congruent. Like Watson and
Hull, the behaviorists with whom he was contemporaneous, Freud tried
to anchor his psychological theory in the consequences of the frustration or satisfaction of *instinctual drive* (*trieb* in German, a concept that
does not translate well but implies a strong behavioral imperative based
on inborn needs of the organism). Sulloway (1979) has persuasively argued that his self-image as a scientist contributed to Freud's choice of
ultimate explanatory units: In his time, as now, a theorist of personality
had reason to worry that he would be seen as insufficiently rigorous
and critical by peers in "hard sciences" such as physics and neuro-
anatomy. Perhaps especially because Freud's professional background
was in medical research, it was important to him that the "science of
psychoanalysis" be rooted in the science of biology, and the biology of
the late nineteenth century was centrally preoccupied with drives. Although I agree with Spezzano (1993) that Freud did, in fact, have an affect theory, it was essentially derivative, emerging from his emphasis on
instinctual drives and their vicissitudes.

Numerous scholars since Freud have for various reasons bemoaned
the consequences of a metapsychology rooted in biological drive.
Intersubjective theorists (e.g., Stolorow & Atwood, 1992), relational
analysts (e.g., Greenberg & Mitchell, 1983), self psychologists (e.g.,
Kohut, 1971), and feminist writers (e.g., Benjamin, 1988), among others, have argued that the biological drive states of the human being are
not the best place to start if we want to comprehend individual psychologies and derive therapeutic principles from our understanding. Still,

there is something to which most of us resonate about the idea of an "id" or an intense state of conflicting needs, longings, and impulses, and the sense of an internal propulsion toward some kind of organic discharge. The Freudian notion of evolving sexual and aggressive tendencies that move from oral to anal to genital expressions was very appealing to several generations of psychoanalytic thinkers, probably in part because it put words around our sense that we are moved by powerful, mostly unconscious forces. If it is not drive that give us the sense of being driven, what is it?

Silvan Tomkins (e.g., 1962, 1963, 1991), the first in a line of generative thinkers researching emotion, argued that it is *affects*. Many post-Freudian therapists and scholars agree (e.g., Izard, 1971, 1979; Rosenblatt, 1985; Greenberg & Safran, 1987; Nathanson, 1990; Spezzano, 1993) and have constructed theories or offered observations based on affect as alternative both to the Freudian drive model and to more current theories that give a privileged position to cognition and behavior, but not to emotion. It has become clear to most therapists in recent decades that in their efforts to understand desire and fear—and a huge part of understanding any individual human being is understanding that person's deepest longings and the anxieties connected with them—they can learn more by assessing someone's affective world than by figuring out at which phase of that person's infancy there was frustration or overgratification of a biological drive.

Having studied with Tomkins, I have been deeply impressed with and influenced by his brilliant and empirically supported case for the existence of nine innate or "hard-wired" affects (Nathanson, 1992): interest–excitement, excitement–joy, surprise–startle, fear–terror, distress–anguish, anger–rage, dissmell (contempt), disgust, and shame–humiliation. I use the term "affect" in a somewhat broader way in this chapter, however, to connote any state of mind and condition of arousal that we have learned to describe as a discrete emotional experience. Thus, I would include under that rubric such diverse phenomena as love, hate, envy, gratitude, boredom, spite, resentment, guilt, pride, remorse, hope, despair, exasperation, tenderness, vindictiveness, pity, scorn, the feeling of being moved or touched, and other emotional conditions.

As psychoanalytic scholarship has progressed, its contributors have pooled considerable knowledge about what happens affectively both in normal development and in psychotherapy. For example, the capacity for affect integration (Socarides & Stolorow, 1984–1985) has been explicated as a maturational accomplishment: Under optimal circumstances, individuals gradually achieve a sense that they are one person with access to diverse affects, none of which threaten the integrity of the self. The concept of "moments" of heightened affect (Stern, 1985; Pine, 1990), based on developmental research rather than speculative *post hoc* reasoning from adult psychopathology (see Chapter Four), has largely replaced theories about wholesale "fixation" at a psychosexual stage because of frustration or overgratification of drives. The capacity to feel and to regulate affect has become a central topic in psychoanalytically influenced empirical research on development and brain physiology, and has led to much recent writing on affect regulation and psychotherapy (e.g., Pally, 1998; Silverman, 1998).

Everyone's individual, idiosyncratic pattern of affective arousal is different. Tomkins could watch someone as he or she talked about current events or other subjects far removed from personal disclosure, and by noting the recurrent patterns of facial affect and the conversational topics with which they were correlated, infer with uncanny accuracy the main features of that individual's unique personality. I imagine that most of us do this unconsciously all the time, probably with less predictive power than Tomkins could typically demonstrate, but nonetheless with a sense that mapping someone's affects and their connection to certain issues is the key to understanding that person's character. (Tomkins was even good at the blind prediction of someone's politics. By seeing a video and noting whether the negative affects on a person's face were distress and disgust or anger and contempt, he could locate him or her as liberal or conservative. His explanation for these correlations made developmental sense, and he was usually right.) In this vein, Kernberg (1997) has noted how therapists process client communications on at least three "channels": (1) verbal communication, (2) body language, and (3) affective transmission, conveyed mostly through facial expressions and tone of voice.

Spezzano (1993) has made a persuasive argument to the effect that the best way to think about character is as "the container and regulator of a person's affects . . . the balance a person has achieved between what is and what might be in his affective life, an expression of his belief about how the greatest sense of well-being can be maintained and how affective pain can best be avoided" (p. 183). This is another way of talking about how people erect a personal shield of defenses against upsetting affects, notably, distress, rage, fear, shame, envy, guilt, and grief. To understand someone, we need to have an appreciation not only of his or her defenses, but also of the affects that are being kept in check by those defenses, and of the affects that are themselves functioning defensively. There are no interview questions that will elicit a person's account of his or her affect pattern, but it is not hard to assess this area. Usually, we evaluate affect subjectively, by assuming that feelings are contagious and noting our own emotional reactions when we are in the presence of a person we want to understand.

AFFECTS IN THE TRANSFERENCE/COUNTERTRANSFERENCE FIELD

For therapists, attention to affect has never been a choice. Patients fill our offices with their feelings; they touch us, inspire us, frustrate us, demoralize us, enrage us, bore us, entertain us, delight us, and surprise us. They weep and laugh and rage and tremble with anxiety. We learn from them about feelings we never knew we had, feelings that may be trivial in our own personal psychological economies but are monumental to some of our clients. The gradual revolution in attitude about countertransference that has characterized the psychoanalytic literature (from a bothersome distraction to be self-analyzed away, to the primary means by which one can understand many clients) is only the articulation of what any honest clinician of any era could hardly avoid noticing. People inject their feelings into their therapists; the most mild, generoushearted practitioner can be turned into a rageful complainer if subjected to a classic paranoid diatribe. Patients create in their treaters conflicts that are parallel to those they have struggled with all their lives, and then they watch to see whether the therapist can model a new way of resolving them. Racker's (1968) useful division of countertransference into concordant ("I'm feeling what the patient was feeling as a child") and complementary ("I'm feeling what the patient's childhood caregivers felt") has allowed therapists to extend their empathy into the affective experience of even the most exasperating clients.

It is often the assessment of one's own affect that allows one to make a critical diagnostic inference. For example, differentiating between an essentially depressive and an essentially self-defeating individual—a discrimination with significant implications for treatment (McWilliams, 1994)—turns on the therapist's noticing that instead of feeling sympathy for a suffering person, he or she is feeling a sadistic inclination to criticize. The realization that one may be dealing with a psychopathic person may come via the therapist's noticing that he or she feels duped or contemptuously bested. The appreciation of a paranoid core under an ostensibly depressive presentation may emerge from the therapist's noting an anxiety-filled fantasy that the patient will file a malpractice suit. We know now that before children can speak, they have highly reliable, exquisitely effective ways of communicating affect nonverbally to their caregivers (Stern, 1985; Beebe & Lachmann, 1988). The residues of those infantile talents in adults express themselves in every interaction. The less effectively a person can communicate emotional suffering in language, the more powerful his or her nonverbal messages tend to be. It is not an accident that the first therapists who conferred dignity on and derived important information from countertransference reactions (e.g., Searles, 1959) were working with more seriously disturbed people, those for whom ordinary speech was often problematic.

Once, I interviewed a teenage boy whose emotional aura was utterly devoid of affect or energized connection with me for most of our interview. Intellectually, I noted that he seemed to be relying on the defenses of withdrawal and omnipotent control. Finally, he began describing, with palpable excitement and in intricate detail, the tortures he regularly inflicted on the family cat. My private emotional reaction was an almost intolerable horror and dread. When he asked at the end of the hour whether I thought he needed treatment, I said yes. "A nice middle-class boy like me?" he teased. "Yes," I said, adding that I thought that without it, he could easily grow up to be a murderer. "You're the only person who has ever understood me," he responded, with deadly sincerity. Nothing in his presentation except the disturbing emotional resonance it created in me had betrayed the degree of sadistic, antisocial ferment at the center of this boy's soul.

What I want to note about this vignette, which is only a particularly dramatic version of what most therapists experience every time they successfully "get" the affective state underlying a client's defensiveness, is that it was via the emotional routes of communication that I "got it" about this boy. I could have derived a hypothesis that he was dangerously antisocial from the objective data: There is considerable research and observation in the field of antisocial behavior attesting to the fact that the torture of animals is associated with adult sadistic behavior toward people. But it was not the intellectual appreciation of these data that allowed me to understand and connect with this client; it was the effect of his emotional state on my own.

I should not conclude this section without a caveat. Although the universality of our central affects (Ekman, 1971, 1980; Tomkins, 1982) suggests that therapists with a disciplined subjectivity and without undue defensiveness (theoretically, those who are "well analyzed" themselves) can find in their own inner emotional lives the basis for resonating to any affective state a patient presents, we all have our limitations. The feelings that are stimulated in us by sitting with a client may not always constitute a complementary or concordant reaction. Therapists must keep in mind the possibility that we are misunderstanding something because it is simply outside our own subjective experience.

To give a nonclinical but germane example: I have a friend who used to exasperate me because she would repeatedly promise to call me on Monday and then would not do so until Wednesday or Thursday. Not only that, when she did call, she would seem genuinely puzzled by my state of aggravation and would explain that she had had so many things going on that the promised time to call had evaporated from her mind. Because it made me angry not to be able to count on her, and because I experienced my own reactive anger as evidence that there was something hostile or avoidant in her behavior, I assumed that her unreliability was expressing negative feelings about me and our friendship.

Not until I listened to a lecture on attention deficit disorder (ADD) in adults (Goldberg, 1998) did I realize my understanding was faulty. (Aptly, the lecture was entitled, "Coming Late May Not Always Be Resistance.") I remembered that my friend had told me she had once been given this diagnosis by a psychiatrist she consulted about her difficulties with remembering and organizing the details of her life. I am a very well-organized person, and without an alternative framework within which to understand her actions, I could not find in myself enough experience with mental disorganization and the inability to prioritize to find empathy with her psychology. With the right "diagnosis" of her behavior, I can now accept that when she says she will phone me on a particular date, I can expect the call within a range of several days. I am sure she is relieved that instead of my grilling her about whether she really wants the friendship, I now handle my hostility by griping about her ADD. Probably, she also feels better understood.

It can be a malignant kind of projection to assume that because one is experiencing certain affects, the person inducing them is (consciously or unconsciously) intending that reaction. As I commented in Chapter Four, one sees this kind of egocentricity frequently: I feel humiliated because I was fired, and I conclude the boss's motive was to shame me. I feel sexually excited, and I conclude that my arouser was trying to be seductive. I feel devastated by the loss of a lover, and I conclude that he wanted to hurt me. I feel frightened by a powerful superior, and I conclude that she was trying to intimidate me. A major difference between such ascriptions and therapists' considered use of their emotional reactions to clients' communications lies in how personally the message is taken. One reason that supervision/consultation groups of therapists are a popular mode of continuing training is that participants can feel out and get some perspective on the emotions that a therapist might be taking too personally. For example, "I'm feeling devalued" can easily turn into "I'm not a very good therapist." The leader and other members, not being in the thick of the transference/countertransference atmosphere, can observe and report on their own more subtle emotional reactions with much less danger of personalizing them.

AFFECT STATES AS PRESENTING PROBLEMS

Some psychopathologies are defined mainly by abnormalities of cognition (e.g., delusions, obsessions, posttraumatic intrusive thoughts), others by abnormalities of behavior (e.g., compulsions, paraphilias, explosivity), others by abnormalities of sensation and perception (e.g., psychogenic pain, anesthesia, hallucination, tunnel vision), and still others by abnormalities of affect (depression and mania, anxiety and panic disorders, phobias). When disturbed affect itself is the presenting clinical problem, the therapist needs to understand its origins and meanings.

Several psychopathologies involving affective disturbance, most notably major depressive and manic states, schizophrenic conditions, and obsessive–compulsive disorders, are currently seen by most researchers as associated with a genetic predisposition. Furthermore, there has been remarkable progress in understanding the neurobiological substrates of certain states of feelings and in finding medications that modify the chemistry of the brain and relieve some of the affective suffering of people with these illnesses. From these data, it is currently commonplace to conclude—and this attitude is reinforced by insurance companies with a financial interest in not supporting psychotherapy—that all one needs to do with people whose affects are problematic is to medicate them. Thus, the hopeless despair of depression, the driven euphoria of mania, the terror in schizophrenic delusions, and the anxiety that fuels obsessions and compulsions are seen as epiphenomenal, symptomatic, and not worth investigating in their own right.

It does not compute, however, that if one of the "causes" is genetic, the cure is simply biological. A genetic predisposition is only that, a predisposition. Not everyone with a probable congenital vulnerability to severe depression becomes severely depressed, just as not everyone with a congenital vulnerability to a heart condition develops cardiac trouble. If the etiology of schizophrenia were simply confined to genetics, then the twin studies suggesting the existence of a constitutional contribution to schizophrenia (Rosenthal, 1971; Gottesman & Shields, 1982) would have found one hundred percent concordance in identical twins when one was found to have that psychosis. The assumed genetic vulnerability, as is true with most "physical" pathologies for which there is a predisposition in the chromosomes, may lay the groundwork for falling ill if certain stresses are suffered (see Zubin & Spring, 1977; Meehl, 1990). We do not get depressed simply because our perverse genes suddenly express themselves; we get depressed because something happens that overwhelms our capacities to cope, making us vulnerable to the activation of any constitutional potential for dysthymia. Without a genetic predisposition, life can still throw us into a depression. With it, we are perhaps more likely to be severely depressed (or manic, or obsessional) and much more subject to subsequent bouts of emotional difficulty. Either way, we need to understand what sets off our potential to be overwhelmed.

People who are on medication for psychological problems with known neurochemical mechanisms still need psychotherapy. They need it in order to feel attached enough to someone who cares about them to have the motivation to keep taking their pills (Frank, Kupfer, & Siegel, 1995). They need it to handle their lives more effectively now that their psychopathology is under better control. They need it to talk about their feelings of being exposed as defective because of their dependency on prescribed drugs. They need it to address the issues that pushed them over some edge that activated their constitutional vulnerability. Sometimes, they need it because they have been told they have a "chemical imbalance," and they wonder why, once the imbalance is rectified, they still suffer so much. I strongly recommend Henry Pinsker's book (1997) on supportive psychotherapy for clinicians who work with medicated patients. Pinsker is unusually astute at naming affects and suggesting interventions that reduce anxiety, support self-esteem, strengthen ego functioning, and improve adaptive skills. I have also been struck by the clinical utility of Gitlin's (1996) beautifully written guide for psychotherapists wanting to know more about psychopharmacology.

I do not feel competent to take a strong position in this area, and I should note that my clinical experience attests more to the utility of some psychotropic medications than to their problematic nature, but I should mention in this context that there is now some evidence (see a discussion of this research and related issues in Wachtel & Messer, 1997) that for at least some people with nonpsychotic depressions, psychotherapy without medication is as effective as psychopharmacology.

Presumably, the therapy process sets in motion an affective reaction that restores neurotransmitters to premorbid levels. Brain chemistry affects emotional experience, but emotional experience also affects brain chemistry. Unmedicated recoveries from depression probably happen through mechanisms such as those discussed by Vaughan (1997) in her highly readable explication of the probable neurochemical *effects* of therapy. I am not surprised that we are now discovering the neurobiology and chemistry of affects. Freud anticipated this, interestingly enough, at least as early as 1926: "In view of the ultimate connection between the things that we distinguish as physical and mental, we may look forward to a day when paths of knowledge and, let us hope, of influence will be opened up, leading from organic biology and chemistry to the field of neurotic phenomena" (p. 231). I am grateful to the new medications for every patient whose suffering they help to reduce, but I am disturbed that these discoveries have been used recently by financially motivated parties to devalue the "talking cure."

EVALUATING THE DIAGNOSTIC MEANING OF AFFECT

Sensitive case formulation has always included, formally or informally, an affect inventory. The obsessive client who cannot feel anger unless it is packaged as moral indignation, the schizoid client who is frightened of tender longings toward real people, the emotionally labile histrionic client, the grim paranoid, the mercurial borderline—almost all our casual diagnostic observation includes implicit assessments of affect (this is true even in the DSM-IV, where criteria for Personality Disorders often include affective elements). In the "mental status" part of the traditional psychiatric examination, there has always been a place for observations about affects: Are they appropriate or inappropriate? Flat? Superficial? Controlled? Can the patient put words to specific feelings or does he or she seem to express feelings via bodily distress? Does the patient feel and express emotions verbally, or are they acted out? The answers to these questions do not just help us to describe someone accurately; they help us formulate ways of helping. There follow some central questions in the evaluation of affect.

Can the Patient Distinguish between Affect and Action?

One should work very differently with someone who can separate affect from action and someone who cannot. Some people can express a hostile fantasy or make a comment about an angry feeling and feel relief from the intensity of a powerful negative reaction. Others seek relief from anger not by verbalizing it but by hitting somebody. For the second type of person, feelings are not well differentiated from the actions that they suggest. Early in my career, I worked with a very angry five-year-old boy whose mother had just had a second child. When he talked about his new brother in a hostile tone, I naively thought it would benefit him to have his anger reflected and validated via a strong statement that would capture the intensity of his feeling. "I bet sometimes you feel so angry toward that baby that you want to throw him out the window!" I announced. Two days later, his mother called me in a state of great alarm. She had found her older son taking his brother out on their second-story porch with the intention to drop him over the railing. What would have been a relieving, emotionally supportive communication to a child who understood that strong feelings can be expressed in fantasy as a *substitute* for behavior was a dangerous message to one who could only experience my words as permission to act out his worst inclinations.

Roger Brooke (1994) gives a similarly disturbing example in the context of discussing people for whom there is no DSM diagnosis that fits, despite obvious pathology.

> One client presented with an inability to experience anger. He knew this was a problem because in those situations when he thought, upon reflection, that it would have been appropriate to be angry he simply "went blank." . . . After some twenty sessions of psychotherapy the therapist . . . made the interpretation that his "going blank" was like his pattern of compliance, and both were ways of avoiding his anger. However, the therapist had missed the point that his patient's problem was not object-related anger—i.e., anger directed towards particular people in specific contexts—but a far more primitive and diffuse rage. His face went pale, he did not speak for the last few minutes of the session and, when he got home, he smashed some of the furniture in his house. Then he went to a bar, got drunk, picked a fight and was arrested by the police. (p. 318)

Can the Patient Represent Affective Experience in Words?

Some people who are not conscious of experiencing feelings act them out, as the aforementioned clients did. Some get sick. One needs to work differently with people who can feel and label affects than with people who cannot. The "alexithymic" ("lacking words for affect") patient, first described by Nemiah and Sifneos (1970; Nemiah, 1978) and later fleshed out by McDougall (1989), cannot be reached by questions such as "How do you *feel?*"—as any clinician who has tried that way of connecting with such a patient can testify. Instead, a therapist trying to help such a client find relief from debilitating somatic expressions of unfelt feeling must first appreciate what McDougall called "inexpressible pain and fears of a psychotic nature, such as the danger of losing one's sense of identity, of becoming mentally fragmented, perhaps of going mad" (p. 25).

Usually, the first way to communicate that appreciation to a client is to focus not on the affects presumed to have given rise to a psychosomatic complaint, but on the affects generated by the complaint itself (e.g., "I can't even imagine how depressing and exasperating it is to be in physical pain most of the time"). In an intake interview with a somatizing patient, if the interviewer moves too quickly to find affects that might be "underneath" the bodily distress, and spends too little time communicating compassion for the client's physical suffering, the somatically disturbed person is all too likely to experience the clinician as accusing him or her of malingering. The client has probably received exactly this message from a series of defeated physicians who have concluded that their patient is a "crock." Consequently, it is critical that a psychotherapist not reinforce the person's experience of having others minimize his or her physical pain.

Many people conventionally diagnosed as obsessive–compulsive personalities are so severely out of touch with what others assume to be natural feelings that the traditional Freudian idea that their emotions are "repressed" is probably a misstatement. Instead of construing such people as suffering from an internal force that keeps a particular emotion from consciousness (an "affect block," as it is sometimes labeled), we may better understand their experience as one of never having learned to represent and elaborate affect. In other words, they do not know "at some level" what they feel and then defend against that feeling; rather, they do not know what they feel. Thus, the therapist's job with such patients is not to penetrate their defenses seeking the warded off feelings but to teach them slowly how to represent unformulated experience in words (see Stern, 1997). Again, it is usually one's countertransference reaction that will indicate whether a given person "knows" at some level what is felt but is keeping it out of the therapeutic relationship because of anxiety or shame, or other negative affect, or whether the person simply has no way to represent internal experience. The former situation will evoke an irritated, impatient countertransference, while the latter engenders feelings of confusion and inarticulateness in the treater. In other words, in the first condition, the therapist feels an affect (e.g., hostility) that presses for discharge; in the second, he or she feels the diffusivity of the unnamed.

How Does the Client Use Affects Defensively?

A related issue is the question of which affects operate in a way that protects a person from feeling other emotional states. It is easy to project onto patients the pattern of one's own affect-maintenance, to attribute to them a similar defensive use of affects, and to assume that what would be therapeutic to oneself is thus therapeutic to others. For example, most therapists have a somewhat depressive cast to their personalities. For them, sadness is often conscious; anger is unconscious. It is therapeutic for such individuals to get access to the hostility and rage beneath their conscious feeling of unhappiness. Theories of psychotherapy that emphasize accessing aggression might be quite appealing to such people, and they might put a lot of confidence in techniques that access or even evoke hostility. If a person with this psychology and its corresponding therapeutic ideology were to treat a patient whose psychological economy worked in an opposite way—for example, a defensively counterdependent man who easily lets anger into consciousness but remains defensively unaware of the more vulnerable emotions of sadness and hurt feelings—the outcome could be disastrous.

A case in point: Stosney (1995) has made a convincing argument on just these grounds, that "anger management training" for abusive partners is misdirected. Contending, with ample evidence, that the problem in batterers is not management of anger but rather the use of anger to defend against fears of abandonment associated with shame, humiliation, and guilt, he has developed a customized and reportedly effective therapeutic strategy emphasizing compassion. (Stosney does not say this, but I infer that the construction of the abuser's problem as the management of anger represents a projection of mental health professionals. If *we* behaved that way, it would mean we did not have our anger under adequately tight rein.) Far from being a "core" affect that a therapist must expose and subject to control, anger is, for many repetitive abusers, a misguided effort to prevent or mitigate much more painful feelings. Batterers seek relief from their pain by projection and acting out, blaming their partners for intolerable emotional states and then attacking them. Stosney's work represents a particularly critical instance of getting it right about affect, with significant consequences for intervention.

A closely related area where therapists frequently get it wrong about affect, again probably because of projection, is the common belief that antisocial individuals are impulsive. Despite massive evidence (see Meloy, 1995) that a significant subgroup of psychopathic people are not at all impulsive—are in fact highly planful and predatory—many of us would rather believe that antisocial aggression represents a loss of control rather than a deliberate strategy to do harm. While the affect that motivates the predatory, "reptilian" psychopath may be rage, it is not a sudden upsurge of anger that is acted out unthinkingly but instead, a cold, calculating fury that is chronically and frontally in consciousness. It is important to understand this if one wants to influence an antisocial person toward behavior change.

Is the Patient's Suffering Related More to Shame or to Guilt?

The affects of shame and guilt have had an interesting history and a special place in psychoanalytic writing. Taken together, they comprise an area in which practitioners' projections and misunderstandings are especially common (a therapist with a guilt-dominated psychology may misunderstand a shame dynamic as guilt-related, and a clinician with tendencies toward shame tends to read indications of guilt as evidence of shame). We all have both, of course, but we differ in which is more central in our respective personalities. Moreover, a particular problem in any of us may represent either guilt or shame. Guilt involves an internal sense of malevolent power, a feeling of deep personal destructiveness and evil. Shame, by contrast, involves a sense of powerless vulnerability, the chronic risk of exposure to the criticism and contempt of others. As Fossum and Mason (1986) have pithily put it, "Guilt is the inner experience of breaking the moral code. Shame is the inner experience of being looked down upon by the social group" (p. vii). Although the degree of a patient's misery does not distinguish a shame from a guilt reaction, because these affects can be equivalently toxic to someone who suffers them, their qualitative differences mean that effective interventions for guilt and shame differ substantially.

Probably because of his own guilt-related dynamics, Freud had little to say about shame but made numerous speculations about guilt. By the middle of the twentieth century, several analytic writers were trying to rectify this imbalance, most notably Helen Merrell Lynd (1958) and

Helen Block Lewis (1971), both of whom wrote extensively about shame and its vicissitudes. In the 1970s, Heinz Kohut and Otto Kernberg published books on pathological narcissism that set off a torrent of psychoanalytic literature on shame-related phenomena. By the 1980s (Tom Wolfe's "Me Decade"—it was not just the analysts who were seeing narcissism and its shame-compensating operations everywhere), the place of shame in our understanding of certain psychological conditions became assured (Lasch, 1984; Kets de Vries, 1989; Morrison, 1989; Nathanson, 1992).

To take only one example of a behavioral propensity that may express either shame or guilt, for which it is critical that the therapist understand which affect is operating, consider the case of pathological perfectionism. Many people are unreasonably perfectionistic, so much so that they are never satisfied with their productions and never finish their work. In the guilt-driven version of this propensity, the compulsion to get everything exactly right expresses a horror that one's destructiveness will slip out of control. Freud's reading of obsessive–compulsive problems put a lot of emphasis on this type of perfectionism. Freudian obsessional patients are chronically afraid their aggressive impulses will erupt, do damage, make a mess. In the shame-driven version of perfectionism, the compulsion expresses the terror of being exposed to the critical scrutiny of others, and exposed not as morally bad but as inadequate, empty, a sham. What Rothstein (1980) called "the narcissistic pursuit of perfection" is a driven determination to appear sinless and flawless, so that one's human limitations are not revealed and others' disdain is avoided.

Naturally, patients who have more shame-related tendencies are not helped by therapists' knee-jerk Freudian assumptions about the guilt-ridden meaning of their perfectionistic curse. Because they represent a serious misunderstanding, interpretations will fall completely flat if they focus on clients' presumed fears that their aggressive impulses will get out of control. Similarly, guilt-dominated perfectionists will not feel the slightest relief from a practitioner who tries to empathize with their presumed worries that they are essentially fraudulent and will be found out. The surface of the vast literature on guilt and shame cannot even be scratched here, but I hope I have addressed the diagnostic issues sufficiently to alert clinical interviewers to the importance of this dimension of affect evaluation. Let me turn now to general comments about the importance of accuracy when one is dealing with a patient's emotional life.

THERAPEUTIC IMPLICATIONS OF GETTING
IT RIGHT ABOUT AFFECT

In the histories of many people who become psychotherapy patients, parents and other caregivers have either (1) neglected the person's feelings, (2) named feelings in a tone of negative judgment (e.g., "You're just feeling sorry for yourself"), (3) punished their children for feelings (e.g., "I'll give you something to cry about!"), or (4) made inaccurate attributions of feeling (e.g., "You're not really jealous—you love your sister!"). The therapist's simply welcoming and being interested in feelings compensates for the first error; naming affects nonjudgmentally mitigates the effects of the second; encouraging safe emotional expression addresses the third; naming feelings accurately helps with the fourth. Perhaps the most challenging of these different correctives is the last. It is not always easy to be accurate. Our individual psychologies set invisible limits on our empathy.

To illustrate, let me mention briefly a client I treated several years ago. This forty-year-old man was the third son of a mother who had wanted a girl so desperately that she put him in dresses until he was almost five and repeatedly told him how deeply his gender had disappointed her. As an adult, although psychologically heterosexual, he kept his distance from women, around whom he was inarticulately uncomfortable. He came to me for help in moving closer to women, hoping to abate his painful loneliness. For a while, he seemed to make progress via my exploring how much anger he carried toward females, anger that appeared in a recurrent transference to me as the mother who saw him as irreparably flawed and disappointing. But then, the therapy seemed to bog down; my naming his anger did not seem to be doing anything for him any more. The treatment process came to life again only when I was able to see that the more driving—and difficult—emotion for him was envy. He hated women for having whatever it was that would have made him acceptable to his mother (see Klein, 1957). He could not enjoy his sexuality because it involved appreciating rather than hating the sexual organs that he lacked. I imagine I am not the first female therapist who took a while to see this dynamic in a man, as most women are more attuned to female envy of male power than to the converse; we need to make an empathic leap to comprehend how central and overwhelming a man's envy of the feminine can be.

I discuss in Chapter Eight how an erotic transference can mean any number of different things about a client's psychology. For now, let me note that it is a relatively frequent experience of mine for a male practitioner in one of my supervision/consultation groups to present the case of a female patient who feels overwhelmed with desire for her therapist and is importuning him to become her lover. His feelings toward her include love, tenderness, and sexual attraction, but they are also becoming tinged with exasperation and anger that she is not letting him do his job—namely, to be a therapist and help her with the problems she came to treatment to address. He wants help with the case from his colleagues and me because his repeated explanations about the importance of observing professional boundaries are falling on deaf ears, and he does not know how to say no in any other way without hurting the client. He is trying to protect her from feeling a devastating rejection of herself and her sexuality; simultaneously, he is struggling not to be seductive, despite the fact that she has succeeded in turning him on.

Typically, in this kind of case presentation, the other therapists in the group find themselves feeling not attracted to or protective of the patient but irritated with her (and often with the presenter). The tender, solicitous feelings the treating clinician describes are notably absent from their emotional responses. Working on the assumption that the group members are feeling something about the interaction that the treater cannot access, we explore the possibility that the patient's affects are not wholly or even predominantly loving; that they instead include considerable hostility, which betrays itself in her implicit effort to disempower the therapist (as is hinted at in his awareness of exasperation that she is keeping him from doing his rightful job). Once the therapist realizes this, he is usually able to help the client find the negative affects that coexist with her love and longing. The acknowledgment by the patient of her hostility and wish to take away her therapist's power over her by asserting her own sexual power (in Freudian language, to castrate him symbolically) makes her feel more fully honest and known, opens the door to her finding positive ways to use her hostility and ambition, and gets the therapy back to the task of understanding her and solving her life problems in realistic ways.

Accuracy about emotional labeling enhances affective and social maturation. Decades ago, Katherine Bridges (1931) mapped out a detailed description of the normal development of the infant's capacity to discriminate and express his or her own affect. Emotional awareness, she observed, begins in the newborn with consciousness of either general contentment or general distress. As the child develops, he or she becomes able to differentiate anger, fear, and sadness from global distress, and then eventually becomes aware of different degrees and tones of each of these (e.g., anger subdivides into irritation, exasperation, rage, fury, and other shades of discontent; contentment subdivides into interest, excitement, joy, surprise, and other positive states). Ideally, this branching-out, increasingly fine-tuned capacity to discriminate and label feeling states continues throughout the lifespan, as we get more and more precise at articulating our emotions to ourselves and others. The pleasure in representing ourselves accurately can enhance self-esteem and feelings of competence even when the emotions in question are painful. It was this phenomenon that inspired one of my colleagues to label herself an "affect junky." She told me she would rather feel *anything,* provided she could name it, than feel numb, detached, confused, or intellectualized. Stephen Sondheim's song "Being Alive" from the musical *Company* captures this state of mind perfectly.

Because many psychotherapy patients have had little help from childhood caregivers in labeling their emotions accurately, they are often further back in the branching-out process than most of us. Some have never had even the most rudimentary feeling states named and accepted. The immediate popularity in different eras of theorists such as Rogers (e.g., 1951), Kohut (1971, 1977), and Miller (1975), who emphasize the therapeutic power of mirroring the patient's emotional state, suggests how widespread is the human need for a witness, namer, and validator of feelings. A significant part of the healing process in any kind of therapy is the practitioner's helping, by naming affects, to foster the patient's sense of mastery over complex and difficult states of arousal.

When therapists name affects, they often presume, in accordance with the Freudian topographical model, that they are "uncovering" feelings that exist already and are kept from consciousness by one or more layers of defense. It is just as likely, and current investigations into affect and its communication suggest that this may be truer, that when we put words to affects, we are implicitly suggesting that the patient should convert his or her current feelings to the emotions we think would be more natural or mature or adaptive. For example, it is a common clinical experience to work with a person who is being mistreated or simply inconvenienced, and who has no conscious sense of anger about it. The therapist asks, "How did you feel when your partner criticized you that way?" and looks skeptical when the patient avoids saying anything about anger. Or the therapist comments, "You must have been at least somewhat irritated when I raised the fee," and interprets any subsequent protestations as a defense against a natural angry response to an increased financial burden.

These interactions are typically construed by the therapist as helping the patient find what he or she already feels but is unable to admit or verbalize. And sometimes, for instance, in situations in which the patient is acting in patently hostile ways while denying negative feelings, such a construction makes the most sense out of the clinical data. But at other times, the patient truly lacks the emotional response the therapist thinks would be natural. In these circumstances, suggesting an affect as a response to whatever stress the patient reports actually influences the person in a new direction of organizing his or her experience. This certainly occurs with alexithymic patients, but it also happens in other people to whom it has never occurred to feel a different way about something.

One patient of mine, a therapist herself, came to a session drowning in guilt after a supervisor had propositioned her. She felt she had been unconsciously seductive, and she was probably right. When I asked whether she had any feelings of anger that her supervisor had used his position of emotional power for sexual purposes, irrespective of her seductiveness, she was able to access (or generate?) enough hostility toward him to counteract somewhat the paralyzing effects of her guilt. She could now use the energy that is inherent in hostility in the service of figuring out what kind of relationship, if any, was now possible with this man. I do not think I "uncovered" her anger. I suspect, instead, that I put the idea in her mind that anger was a reasonable emotional response. Analytic therapists do not like to see themselves as actively suggesting or educating, but in the affective realm, we may do more of that than we admit.

Affects are motivators. By attaching a feeling to an experience, we often find the emotional resources to solve a problem that had seemed previously hopeless. This process can happen on a social as well as an individual level. Political leaders typically try to connect pressing circumstances or events with emotional reactions (excitement, pride, fear, anger) because those affects will energize people toward a social goal. The feminist movement of the early 1970s was significantly catalyzed by Jane O'Reilly's (1972) depiction of how an emotional "click" would register in the sensorium of a hitherto uncomplaining housewife at the moment when a previously absorbed insult was reformulated as a cause for righteous anger.

Affects, when adequately expressed and understood, also accomplish developmental goals. The best illustrator of this function is the role of grief. In the normal mourning process, nature seems to have endowed us with a capacity to make emotional peace with the inevitable disappointments of life. At every life stage that symbolically bids goodbye to one's previous role, at every loss, at every instance of realizing our limitations, our inability to have it all, we need to accomplish a piece of mourning if we are to avoid regression or psychological rigidity (see Judith Viorst's [1986] eloquent popularization of psychoanalytic ideas on this topic in *Necessary Losses*). Oddly, because he did not develop his ideas on the topic systematically afterward, it is Freud who first suggested the importance of this function. In 1917, building on Abraham's (1911) seminal research on depression, Freud wrote the evocative masterpiece "Mourning and Melancholia," in which he argued, among other things, that grief and depression are in a sense opposites: When one reacts to a loss with grief, the *world* seems emptier for the absence of the person mourned; when one reacts with depression, the *self* feels diminished. Much of what we call psychotherapy consists in the conversion of depressive reactions into mourning so that the developmental process can become unstuck, and the client can grieve and move on.

Anxiety, not sadness, was at the center of Freud's implicit affect theory. Not having a particularly depressive sensibility himself, Freud was naturally preoccupied with a feeling that was more central to his experience (see Stolorow & Atwood, 1979, 1992). His interest in the "traditional" neuroses (hysterical conditions, obsessive–compulsive disorders, and phobic reactions) also inclined him toward an emphasis on anxiety and its containment or relief, since anxiety is more central to those disturbances. Both his etiological premises and his technical recommendations depended on the assumption that anxiety is the core pathogenic affect. In contrast, most contemporary therapists have been increasingly impressed with the importance of other negative affects— especially grief, guilt, shame, and envy—both in terms of symptom formation and in terms of therapeutic interventions.

With respect to grief, Stark (1994), for example, understands much psychopathology in terms of unmourned experience. Such a formulation applies with particular salience to the personality disorders. Accordingly, she construes psychotherapy as essentially a grieving process, in which a compassionate other helps the patient face up to painful realities that have been previously regarded as evidence of his or her personal deficits. As I mentioned in Chapter One, Stark incisively observes that the first months or years of therapy are generally taken up with clients' gradual assimilation of the fact that their problems are not their fault. Then during the subsequent months or years, clients come to terms with the fact that even though their troubles are not their fault, they are the only ones who can do something about them. This gradual accommodation to painful reality involves giving up and mourning all their fantasies that some omnipotent good object (perhaps the therapist) will fix things. It is analogous to the process we all go through, in optimal development, in which we come to terms with the unfairness of life and learn to rely on our own activity to solve its inescapable problems.

SUMMARY

I introduced this chapter with some commentary on the history of attention to affect in both psychoanalytic theory and clinical practice. Then, I discussed how, in the transference and countertransference matrix of clinical involvement, a therapist tries to evaluate affect, keeping in mind that one cannot be certain that one's disciplined subjectivity is always picking up the patient's true emotional state. In the case of those psychopathologies essentially defined by disturbances of affect, I argued that psychotherapy is needed even when medications can transform affective experience. In addressing how to understand someone's emotional life, I considered the capacity to differentiate affect from action, the ability to represent emotional states in words, the defensive uses of affect, and the discrimination of shame from guilt. Finally, I discussed the therapeutic implications of understanding the workings of emotion, both in specific individuals and instances, and in general, as in the appreciation of psychotherapy as a grieving process.

❦

CHAPTER SEVEN

Assessing Identifications

ONE does not have to be a mental health professional to know that a central aspect of any person's psychology involves the people who were his or her major love objects and models. In intake interviews, clients will almost always readily discuss the people in their backgrounds to whom they see themselves as similar, the people they have wanted to emulate, and the people they have tried at all costs *not* to be like. One of the main limitations of standard descriptive diagnosis is that any given behavior may mean remarkably different things psychologically, depending on the individual with whom that behavior is consciously or unconsciously identified.

There is probably no such thing as a behavior or attitude that is not influenced by identifications, and what those identifications are can vary greatly. A woman who habitually criticizes and carps may be unconsciously trying to be like her beloved but overcontrolling grandmother, or she may be reassuring herself that she is *not* like her passive and negligent mother, who let others walk all over her. Or both. A man who is irritatingly "rational" about things that other people experience as emotionally loaded may be identifying with a hyperintellectualized father, or with the cerebral high school teacher who set an inspiring counterexample to a father who would explode over trifles. Or he may have had younger siblings, whose emotionality was labeled babyish, with whom he is determinedly counteridentified. Or if his mother was the emotive one in the family, he may be reassuring himself that he is not female. To be optimally therapeutic, practitioners need to know the identificatory meanings behind their clients' attitudes and behavior.

Typically, in an early interview, one asks the client about his or her mother and father or other primary caregivers: Are they alive? If not, when did they die, and of what? If alive, how old are they? What are (were) their occupations? What are (were) their respective personalities like, and how were they as parents? Sometimes one learns a fair amount from inquiring about which one the client resembles, and in what ways. It is also important to ask whether there were other significant influences on the interviewee as he or she was growing up. Sometimes it will emerge that a teacher or clergy person or camp counselor or therapist or friend had a powerful influence because of the patient's identification with that person. People are conscious of many aspects of their identifications. Yet a whole different level of information about an individual's internalizations may come through less conscious, less verbal means.

IDENTIFICATIONS SUGGESTED
BY TRANSFERENCE REACTIONS

In a clinical interview, the quickest way to assess a person's primary identifications is to feel out the overall tone of the transference. Sometimes its manifestations are subtle, as in the benign sense of connectedness one gets with a person raised by loving parents, whose generosity of spirit has been internalized and permeates the intake session. Or, equally subtly but less gratifyingly, the transference tone comes through in the therapist's vague sense of being devalued, as when a client asks more than a moderate number of questions about one's training, provoking the tentative hypothesis that he or she has identified with someone skeptical or distrusting.

Sometimes an initial transference is more startling and stark. A colleague of mine recently reported evaluating a woman who had seen several previous practitioners in an effort to deal with her problem managing anger. All her prior therapists had blundered in one way or another, she explained, mainly by failing to understand her adequately. She was worried that my colleague would similarly disappoint her. Appreciating her sensitivity to being misunderstood, he tried hard in his initial remarks not to make any premature attributions, but at the end of the first interview he commented, "It usually takes me a few sessions to develop a preliminary understanding of someone. It might take me a bit longer with you because your psychology seems rather complicated." The client went into a rage on the grounds that the term "complicated" was an evasive way of calling her crazy. (One sees here a familiar combination of accurate perception—she was not wrong in sensing that the therapist felt her problems were severe—and skewed interpretation of attitude, in that the therapist was not feeling critical and devaluing toward her.) It was natural for the therapist to infer that this woman had internalized at least one authority whose primary attitude was intensely critical.

Sometimes people are completely unaware of their similarity to an early love object. One woman I interviewed spent a good part of our first meeting complaining about her mother's intrusive, controlling, and unreasonably finicky attitude. I felt very sympathetic to her situation as the child of someone so hard to please. We seemed to have made a good connection, and my countertransference to her was quite warm until she was about to leave my office. At that point she looked with unmistakable consternation at the paintings on the wall and straightened them out so that there was no unevenness in the way they hung. "There," she said. "Now you won't have to be embarrassed about how your office looks."

IDENTIFICATION, INCORPORATION, INTROJECTION, AND INTERSUBJECTIVE INFLUENCING

Freud (1921) wrote about two kinds of identificatory processes, an early, relatively unconflicted "anaclitic" object love (from the Greek word "to lean on," implying straightforward dependency) and a later process that eventually became known as "identification with the aggressor" (A. Freud, 1936). The former is a benign phenomenon in which a child—or adult, for that matter, but these processes are both more conspicuous and more consequential for personality formation in children—loves a caregiver and wants to have the qualities that make that person lovable. When a little boy explains, "I want to be like Mommy because she is sweet," he is expressing an anaclitic identification. Identification with the aggressor, contrastingly, occurs in upsetting or traumatic situations and operates as a defense against fear and the sense of impotence. It is more automatic and less subjectively voluntary, but if one were to put words to the process they would be, "Mother is terrifying me. I can master this terror with the fantasy that I'm the mother, not the terrified, helpless child. I can reenact this scene with myself as the instigator and thereby reassure myself that I will not be the victim this time." Weiss and Sampson and their colleagues (Weiss, Sampson, & the Mount Zion Psychotherapy Research Group, 1986) refer to this process as "passive-into-active transformation."

Freud tended to write and speculate in greater detail about the latter kind of identification, not because it was more common, but because it was more unconscious, problematic, and at variance with commonsensical, rationalistic, and behavioral explanations of behavior. His description of the identification that results from the oedipal situation is basically an identification-with-the-aggressor explanation, although in healthy family situations, the aggression is not so much in the parent as projected there by the child. In the classical oedipal triangle, the child longs for one parent, feels competitive with the other, becomes worried (because feelings and actions are not yet fully separate in the child's mind) that his or her aggression is dangerous, becomes afraid of retaliation from the object of the aggression, and then resolves this anxiety-filled predicament by a decision to be like the person of whom he or she is afraid ("I can't get rid of Daddy and have Mommy, but I can be like Daddy and have a woman like Mommy"). This scenario throws light on many diverse psychological phenomena, including, for example, the persistence of triangular themes in literature, the anxieties and depressive reactions people commonly suffer when they have attained some personal triumph, and the tendency for children between three and six to have nightmares in which they are threatened by monsters of their own aggressive imaginings.

For a period of time in the mid-twentieth century, oedipal, identification-with-the-aggressor formulations became such a popular way of understanding identification that research psychologists were spending considerable energy demonstrating the existence of a nonconflictual type of identification. Sears and his colleagues (e.g., Sears, Rau, & Alpert, 1965), after designing a number of ingenious experiments that elicited an automatic and emotionally uncomplicated type of identification, coined the term "modeling" to contrast this process with the anxiety-filled, defensively motivated oedipal scenario sketched out by Freud. Interestingly, the notion of modeling is quite similar conceptually to Freud's observations about anaclitic attachments.

Anyone who has watched preschoolers play knows how startling it is to see them enact every detail of a parent's tone and gesture. Some identification, especially the kind seen in young children, looks like a kind of "swallowing whole" of the person being taken in. Even in older people—for example, a college student who has become enamored of a particular mentor, or a cult member emulating a revered guru—one sometimes sees such a wholesale incorporation of the esteemed object that the person identifying seems to have disappeared and become a clone of his or her idol. An idealizing admirer can pick up the way someone walks, talks, laughs, sighs, and eats spaghetti. In other instances, identification strikes one as more nuanced and subjectively voluntary: The identifier takes on some features of the object and rejects others. Most of us can readily describe both the aspects of ourselves that represent our wish to be like a childhood influence and the aspects that represent our resistance to such identifications.

In post-Freudian psychoanalytic writing, there is a long scholarly tradition, fed by the distress of therapists confronting the maladaptive identifications of their patients, of trying to understand the development of normal identificatory processes. In 1968, Roy Schafer described a progression in children from a swallowing-whole type of assimilation of a caregiving person (cf. Jacobson, 1964) through stages of greater and greater discrimination and reflection, approaching finally a seasoned process of *identification*, in which the object is appreciated as a complex, differentiated Other, whose qualities are appropriated in a way that feels to the child more selective and voluntary. While two-year-olds simply march around with their mother's pocketbook, children in the oedipal years can comment engagingly about just which qualities of which parent they want to adopt.

Some writers have used the term "identification" very broadly; others, like Schafer, have tried to differentiate between earlier incorporation and later forms of taking in the qualities of others. Empirical evidence now suggests that the development of internal representations of caregivers proceeds simultaneously with the development of internal representations of self (Bornstein, 1993), and that these representations of self and other evolve in hierarchical stages, influencing a child's perceptions, expectations, and behaviors (Horner, 1991; Schore, 1997; Wilson & Prillaman, 1997). In contemporary psychoanalytic writing, the term "introjection" is most commonly used (probably because it can be neatly contrasted with its counterpart process, projection) for the kinds of internalization that predate more mature identificatory processes. The internalized images of people important to the developing child are thus called *introjects*. As the internalization process matures from presumably unreflective mimicry to discriminating, subjectively voluntary efforts to take on certain specific features of someone else's personality, it looks less introjective and more deliberately identificatory.

The identification *process* seems quite uniform across families and cultures. The *content* of an identification can be either benign or deeply problematic. When one's earliest internalizations are maladaptive, they present grave difficulties for therapy later because of their preverbal, automatic nature. In her doctoral research, my former student, Ann

Rasmussen (1988), interviewed women who had been repeatedly and viciously abused by their lovers and spouses. Her subjects were the kinds of people who typically exhaust the reserves of workers in women's shelters: They kept going back to their abusers. During one meeting, the two-year-old son of her interviewee made a Play-Doh representation of a scar, which he proudly stuck to his cheek and showed off to his mother and her guest. His introjection process was normal, but the content of his effort to be like his mother boded badly for his future.

The original psychoanalytic literature on this topic concentrated on the child's acquisition of parental characteristics as if the child's development were dynamic and the parent's influence were relatively static. More recent psychoanalytic research and theorizing about development (e.g., Brazelton, Koslowski, & Main, 1974, Brazelton, Yogman, Als, & Tronick, 1979; Trevarthan, 1980; Lichtenberg, 1983; Stern, 1985, 1995; Beebe & Lachmann, 1988; Greenspan, 1981, 1989, 1997) addresses identificatory processes from a more intersubjective standpoint, emphasizing the mutual influences that the child and caregiver exert on each other. In fact, the more we learn about how people develop their sense of individual identity, the more back-and-forth the process of identification seems to be: An infant takes in characteristics of its mother, who changes to adapt to her particular baby, who reinternalizes the changed mother, and so on.

The existence of this intersubjective "dance" (cf. Lerner, 1985, 1989) is one reason we cannot assume that an internalized object is equivalent to a living person. The father I originally identified with was the omnipotent, omniscient father of my earliest idealizing perceptions, not the man I grew to appreciate as an adult, who was both fragile in his self-esteem and uncertain in his understanding. Accidents of history can also affect the nature of internalizations. I once treated a young man for a pervasive aloofness. All his relationships, including his connection with me, seemed cold and rejecting. His explanation for his tendency to distance from people was that his mother was a "human refrigerator," incapable of warmth. In our initial interviews, I found him a difficult and perplexing client, incapable of mutuality to the extent that he could not even be engaged in recounting his personal history. I asked his permission to interview his mother and braced myself to deal with an automaton. To my astonishment, she was not only warm but also deeply loving and concerned for her son. It emerged in her account of his childhood that during the first months of his life, she had had a serious contagious illness and had been forbidden to touch or hold him.

Other relatives had given him minimal custodial care. The refrigerator mother he had internalized was nothing like the flesh-and-blood parent who wept in my office about his rejection of all her efforts to reach him.

One important part of a diagnostic formulation is the assessment of how primitive or mature are the client's identificatory processes. Kernberg (1984), one of the more articulate diagnosticians in a long line of therapists who have known the value of asking patients about their early objects, has argued for the specific utility of asking an incoming patient to describe his or her parents and other significant influences. Generally speaking, it is diagnostic of individuals at the borderline and psychotic levels of psychological organization to describe others in global, holistic ways that emphasize either their overall goodness or their irredeemable badness, while people in the neurotic and healthy ranges give balanced and multidimensional accounts of people (cf. Bretherton, 1998). Information of this sort is important to the therapist in choosing whether to conduct treatment along the lines of a supportive, expressive, or uncovering model (Kernberg, 1984; Rockland, 1992a, 1992b; McWilliams, 1994; Pinsker, 1997).

Both of the aforementioned clients, the woman with the anger problem and the aloof young man, depicted their parents in unidimensional ways. When listening to such descriptions, the interviewer typically feels at a loss for any sense of what the described person is really like. The object presented comes across as either a saint or a Satan, not a struggling human being trying to cope with being a parent as well as possible given whatever handicaps his or her own personal history and current circumstances have created. Both of these illustrative clients were appropriately diagnosable as in the borderline range developmentally; typologically, the woman was organized in a predominantly paranoid way, and the man was more schizoid. The combination of paranoid and borderline dynamics that she presented required a supportive stance from the therapist, whereas he responded well to expressive therapy.

But even people who are quite mature psychologically can have areas in which they have unreflectively put certain objects in all-good or all-bad categories. Hysterically organized clients, for example, have the reputation for being quite impressionistic about people, even when they are otherwise capable of astute and incisive insights (Shapiro, 1965). Similarly, high-functioning depressive people tend, like more disturbed depressive individuals, to be all-or-nothing in their identifications, often having only negative perceptions about themselves and nothing but good to say about others (Jacobson, 1971). In hysterically oriented and histrionic clients, this tendency to idealize or devalue defends against perceptions that stimulate fears of being overwhelmed or injured; in depressive ones, it protects the hope that by association with good objects, the badness in their own soul can be counteracted.

CLINICAL IMPLICATIONS
OF UNDERSTANDING IDENTIFICATIONS

Data about internalizations, especially those that have an all-good or all-bad flavor, have significant implications for psychotherapy above and beyond the general question of conducting supportive versus expressive versus uncovering treatment. First, they cue the interviewer about how to try to make an initial connection with a patient. A good general rule is for the therapist to find ways, within standard professional practice, to exemplify how he or she differs from the patient's pathogenic internalized objects. If a person reports that a parent was unremittingly self-centered, the therapist needs to demonstrate an altruistic sensibility. If the internalized parent is critical, the accepting aspects of a therapy relationship require special emphasis. If the introject is seductive, the therapist must be especially careful about professional boundaries. These sensitive responses will not prevent the patient from eventually experiencing the therapist as like the internalized objects, but they will make it more likely that once such transferences appear, the client will appreciate the difference between his or her projections and the features of the therapist that contradict what has been projected.

Second, as implied in the foregoing paragraph, these data give the practitioner advance notice of the nature of the main transferences that will appear in treatment. Identifications are powerful and driving psychological forces. No amount of determined kindness from a therapist will prevent a victim of childhood abuse from going through the experience of feeling that he or she is about to be (or has been) abused by him or her. No demonstration of acceptance is adequate to ward off the conviction of immanent rejection held by patients who have internalized a rejecting object. Nor would it be advantageous to most clients if a therapist's efforts to be discriminated from the internalized objects were successful over time. People come to therapy precisely because experiences that "should" have counteracted the expectations laid down in their childhoods have failed to have that effect. They need to project onto the therapist the internalized figures that keep compromising their growth and satisfaction, and then learn to relate to them in a manner different from the one they adopted in childhood. Freud (e.g., 1912), reflecting on transference and its therapeutic potential, was fond of commenting that one cannot fight an enemy *in absentia.*

Third, understanding the cast of characters that have lived in the mind of one's client and what each of them means to him or her is critical to devising strategies to help. Sometimes it is the only avenue down which one can move to a position of influence. Some years ago, I worked with a man who was chronically and relentlessly suicidal. When his bipolar illness did not have him completely in its grip, he was a delightful, creative, and highly effective clergyman, husband, and father. My sessions with him when he was not acutely depressed were riveting and moving, and they were also productive in the sense that he valued what he was learning about himself and was able to make numerous positive changes in his behavior.

When his depressive feelings overcame him, however, he could find no reason to live, despite the pleadings of a substantial number of people who loved him and relied upon him. He had a suicide kit at home, a cache of pills more than adequate to do him in, and all my efforts at negotiating with him to get rid of the tools for his destruction only elicited from him the comment that if I insisted that he give up the means to kill himself, he would be glad to lie to me and say he had done it, but he had no intention of sacrificing the sense of ultimate control and autonomy that his suicide kit gave him. Understandably, he gave me several sleepless nights, and more than once, I encouraged him to hospitalize himself when his wish to die seemed palpably stronger than his interest in living.

This client's suicidal intentions were highly overdetermined. His family history suggested a clear genetic contributant to bipolar illness. In addition, he had been unrelentingly criticized, controlled, and physically abused by his mother, leaving him with the internal conviction that he deserved punishment, and that his inherent badness would ultimately earn him rejection by anyone who really got to know him. When he was a young child, his only escape from his mother's mistreatment was running away, something he did in large and small ways from the time he could locomote. It comforted him to know he could exit the world if life became unbearable. In his mind, his suicide kit represented the equivalent of the escape routes he had used as a child. He had also been sternly socialized never to express or even acknowledge the feeling of anger. He consequently experienced any aggressive feelings as part of his badness, and he would berate himself for even trivial instances where he felt his unwitting hostility or selfishness had hurt someone.

His self-esteem had been damaged by a family that cared more about how he looked to others than about how he felt internally, and his sense of efficacy had been crippled by his powerlessness to influence either his mother's tirades or his father's passive–aggressive, alcohol-contaminated responses to them.

I had tried, as had his psychiatrist and several emotionally astute relatives and friends, to confront his stubborn suicidality by making his anger more conscious, by analyzing his irrational but understandable conviction that he was bad, by calling his attention to his wishes to pay his mother back for her abuse of him by mortifying her with his suicide, by realistically looking at what it would mean to his wife and three children if he killed himself, and by exploring his Tom Sawyeresque fantasies of what people would feel and say at his funeral. I tried to get him to pay attention to the transference, to explore how he imagined it would affect me if he died, and to find the hostility in that and express it in less self-destructive ways. None of this had much effect.

One thing that did engage him, however, was an exploration of his identification with his father. A critical feature of this client's history was that his own father had committed suicide after a particularly wounding remark by his wife. My patient had looked desperately to this man to protect him from his mother's attacks and to give him an alternative model of how to be an adult. It emerged that he deeply admired his father for killing himself, as it was the only time he had ever seen anyone get the last word with his mother. He regarded the suicide as the consummate grand gesture, an irreversible "Fuck you!" to a woman who had acted tyrannically toward both her husband and her boy. One of the compelling attractions of suicide to him was its meaning as a masculine rejection of feminine dictatorship.

Once we had made this connection, we could look together at whether his father's suicide had actually been an act of courage or whether he had simply needed to see it that way, in preference to confronting the painful realization that his father was so weak and demoralized that he let his wife's mistreatment destroy him. Eventually, this patient went through a kind of epiphany in which he realized he was furious at his father for abandoning him. At that point, he could appreciate emotionally rather than just intellectually what he would be doing to his children if he deprived them of his existence. He could also think about how another man might have responded to his mother's behavior and imagine a much less self-destructive version of masculine strength. His identification with his father was diminished, and his emotional readiness to take in the qualities of other male figures was enhanced.

Finally, it is important for therapists to understand primitive and unidimensional internal presences because the appreciation of complexity and contradiction in others and in the self is such a central aspect of psychological maturity and personal serenity. That appreciation remains an important overall goal in long-term psychotherapy. The clinician thus tries to help modulate a patient's all-good and all-bad images, to bring into awareness the positive features of a hated object and the negative aspects of a revered one, to find love alongside hate and hate where the person has been conscious only of love. Eventually, in effective therapy, stark and unidimensional images are replaced with realistic perceptions of the strengths and weaknesses of any individual human being. People who become more accepting of the emotional and moral complexity of others also become more accepting of their own assets, liabilities, and contradictions.

This principle of modifying all-bad and all-good internalized images applies even to people who have been savagely mistreated by early authorities who seem nothing short of monstrous to the therapist. People cling to their internalized objects, however bad they are, in the same way that abused children cling to their abusive caretakers. When a therapist joins a client in consigning a parent to the category of "bad," the inevitable fact that the client loved that parent is not being let into consciousness and embraced as part of the self. The therapist has colluded with a disavowal of an important part of the patient's personality. Abused clients need to find their anger at having been damaged, to grieve their tragic histories, and eventually to appreciate that the perpetrators of their injuries were damaged human beings, usually with horrific histories of their own. They need to remember that they both loved and hated their abusers (Terr, 1992, 1993; Davies & Frawley, 1993).

CLINICAL POSSIBILITIES WHERE COUNTERIDENTIFICATION PREDOMINATES

The patient who is determined to be the polar opposite of a destructive parent or caregiver is a familiar clinical phenomenon. I know many people, both among my clients and among my friends and colleagues, whose capacity to take a counteridentificatory position clearly saved them from the worst possible consequences of a difficult history. Research on the sequellae of child abuse (e.g., Haugaard & Reppucci, 1989) has established that even though it is common for abusers to have been the victim of an abusive parent themselves, it is also true that having a brutal childhood does not destine one to be a brute. Many maltreated people have reared their sons and daughters humanely with the help of a powerful internal determination not to recreate their parent's transgressions. Counteridentification can make the difference between emotional devastation and the self-esteem that comes from resisting internal pressures to submit to a self-defeating family pattern.

One problem with counteridentification, however, is that it tends to be total and uncompromising. A friend of mine holds her hypochondriacal mother in such contempt that she avoids medical treatment even when ill. Another acquaintance has been so determined not to be like his alcoholic father that he became a moralistic teetotaler whose children could not resist the temptation to rebel by experimenting with drugs. Therapists are often confronted with clients who cannot consider changing their behavior in a positive direction because the object with whom they are counteridentified used to act that way at times. A woman I know lives in chronic clutter and disorder because her father's second wife, whom she experienced as cold and rejecting, had a passion for neatness and organization. Despite the self-defeating and illogical nature of her position, this accomplished, intellectual woman explains that she cannot clean up her act because it would make her feel too much like her stepmother. To her, being orderly means being cold. (It may have been patients like this that propelled the behavioral movement in psychotherapy to develop a cognitive dimension: Too many people were not doing their homework because it made them feel like someone they hated, about whom they nurtured powerful but irrational attitudes.)

These dynamics are important to understand if the therapist is to avoid the frustration of exploring avenues of change that repeatedly encounter a stubborn resistance. Sometimes a relatively mild observation (e.g., "Because your stepmother was both orderly and cold, you've assumed that to be orderly means to be cold") can liberate a client from the automatic posture of counteridentification. Sometimes it is necessary to make interpretations that have more punch (e.g., "You're so afraid of being like your stepmother that you reject even her good qualities" or "You prefer your disorganization, even though it's obviously self-destructive, to giving your stepmother—who is now dead—the satisfaction that you're like her in any way!"). Often, one cannot make headway with actions that are determined by counteridentification until they appear in the transference ("You're getting to sessions late and cheating yourself of the time you pay for—all because you're experiencing me as an orderly person like your cold stepmother, whom you have to defy at any cost").

Sometimes one can take advantage of a counteridentification to help a person change in a desired direction. A potent antidote to a maladaptive behavior is the therapist's exposure of its meaning as an identification with an early object from whom the patient has earnestly striven to be different. A woman I worked with, who had found her father's grandiose, manic, controlling style unbearable, had made every conscious effort to behave counter to his example. She took pains to be sensitive to others, to allow them their space, to be sure her own agenda never overwhelmed those of the people to whom she was close. She came to me for help with, among other things, the symptom of not being able to manage money well. In particular, she could not resist any pressure from her partner to spend more than they could afford, something she attributed to her general compliance—that is, her counteridentification with her controlling father. It was when we unearthed the fact that her behavior in the financial area was in subtle ways very much *like* her father's, in that he had never been able to resist throwing money around in the service of demonstrating his power, that she was able to put her determination to be different from him into the service of economizing.

On the topic of identification and counteridentification, I cannot resist mentioning the dissertation research of my colleague Kathryn Parkerton (1987). She was interested in whether analysts grieve during or after the termination phase with their analysands, and in pursuing this question, she interviewed ten very experienced practitioners in her area. In the service of getting relevant information, she asked them about many practices related to ending treatment. Did they become more self-disclosing in the final weeks of therapy? Did they ever accept gifts from patients at the end of the work? Did they discourage or encourage the person's relating to them as a colleague or friend once the treatment was over? Did they keep in touch with former analysands? Did they send them Christmas cards? Did they encourage them to come back for "tune-ups" at some future time?

These ten analysts turned out to be all over the map with respect to whether they mourned the end of an analysis. One woman denied any feelings of sadness, explaining that she felt an exhuberant sense of "Bon voyage" and the pleasant anticipation of getting to know a new client. A male analyst confessed that he suffered terribly, going through all the Kübler-Ross stages in relation to each patient who "graduated." Moreover, the subjects varied widely in their answers to the specific questions. Not only were they strikingly diverse, but also—most interesting to me—they all believed that their particular set of rules and practices comprised the "classical" or "accepted" standards of psychoanalytic behavior! What their convictions actually turned out to correlate with were their own analysts' practices: They either handled termination exactly as their own therapist had handled it or in the polar opposite way. They all had rationales for their technical choices, but one suspects that the identification came first and the explanations later.

ETHNIC, RELIGIOUS, RACIAL, CULTURAL, AND SUBCULTURAL IDENTIFICATIONS

Even in the current cultural climate, where issues of diversity have been raised much more than they were during the time of my own training as a therapist, it probably cannot be overemphasized that therapists need to appreciate the ethnic, religious, racial, class, cultural, and subcultural identifications of their clients. A plea for such understanding does not mean that therapists must become experts ahead of time on all the possible backgrounds from which their patients may come (though, as with anything else, the more general knowledge one has, the better); it means that we all must be attentive to the possible implications of identifications very different from our own (Sue & Sue, 1990; Comas-Díaz & Greene, 1994; Foster, Moskowitz, & Javier, 1996). Even the Western notion of an individualized self, however automatically those of us raised in this culture assume such a construct, is not a ubiquitous aspect of human psychology (Roland, 1988). Nevertheless, the phenomenon of identification as a critical developmental process seems universal.

Nothing in the DSM captures the importance for an effective therapeutic connection of understanding how Irish families tend to socialize people to control affect, while Italian ones socialize them to vent it, and what kinds of shame or guilt may overcome people when their actions contravene the messages of their cultures of origin. The kinds of questions explored in *Ethnicity and Family Therapy* (McGoldrick, Giordano, & Pearce, 1996) have had inestimable value for therapists, whether or not they practice a family system model of treatment. Likewise, Lovinger's (1984) *Working with Religious Issues in Therapy* has made it easier for therapists to understand the psychological implications of the contrast between Protestant guilt about *acting* on one's inevitably selfish feelings and Catholic guilt about *having* selfish feelings. When Grier and Cobbs (1968) wrote *Black Rage*, they sensitized a whole generation of Caucasian therapists to the implications of being African-American. More recently, Nancy Boyd-Franklin (1989) has usefully summarized decades of work on black subcultures in *Black Families in Therapy*.

Sometimes it is more important to know that someone is Ukrainian than to know that he or she suffers from a dysthymic disorder. Because a solid working alliance is a necessary condition of doing psychother-apy, those understandings that make an alliance possible are more criti-cal to the success of any individual treatment than the therapist's so-phistication about the dynamics of a specific symptom. When one practices in an area containing an ethnic population considerably differ-ent from one's own, it is important to pursue available knowledge about working with people from that group. Studies over the past two decades (e.g., Acosta, 1984; Trevino & Rendon, 1994) demonstrate that with rather brief training, therapists can reduce the frustrations— and consequent premature terminations—of minority clients who are trying to make themselves understood by therapists from the dominant culture.

If one is unfamiliar with the psychological implications of some-one's coming from a particular ethnic, racial, or cultural background and cannot find good material on the topic, one should simply ask the patient for education about the values and assumptions of his or her group. Not only does such an inquiry make the critical point that there are no conversational taboos in psychotherapy (in contrast to most so-cial settings, where racial, ethnic, and sexual-orientation differences among people are privately noted but rarely discussed), it has been my experience that clients are pleased to be asked, appreciative of a thera-pist's genuine curiosity about their heritage, and generous with their knowledge. In fact, the experience of teaching one's therapist can have a nice counteractive effect on the patient's feeling that the role of the person seeking help is a one-down position in which the therapist has expertise and the client has only ignorance.

When misunderstandings inevitably happen in a treatment between therapist and client of different backgrounds, therapists are well ad-vised not to jump to textbook conclusions about the meaning of the dif-ficulty, but to draw out the patient about his or her experience, expecta-tions, and assumptions. A cautionary area in which ethnic differences may determine what is therapeutic versus what is destructive, and where it is hard not to make mistakes, involves instances when the cli-ent brings a gift to the therapist. Cultures vary widely in their attitudes toward gifts, in the functions that gift giving performs, and in their members' expectations about the proper ways gifts are to be received. Standard psychoanalytic practice has always been for therapists to turn down gifts—with warmth and tact, but nonetheless with the clear communication that in a psychotherapy relationship, transactions are expected to be in words, not acts. It has been a good general rule for therapists to assume that when a patient feels impelled to bring a present to the therapist, something is being expressed in an action that should be converted into a verbalization and then understood together. The old adage "Analyze, don't gratify" (in this case, do not gratify the ostensibly generous impulse of the gift giver—find out what is being expressed with the gift) has become lodged in the superego of a whole generation of dynamically inclined therapists. In fact, impassioned controversies about the theory of psychotherapy have been known to swirl around the question of simple transactions such as whether it is ever appropriate for a clinician simply to accept a gift without any comment other than "thank you" (e.g., Langs & Stone, 1980).

For a therapist to turn down a small gift—however graciously—from someone strongly identified with caregivers in a subculture in which gift giving is expected in both personal and business transactions, is to invite a therapeutic crisis. No matter how tactfully educated, the client is likely to be wounded in his or her effort to identify with respected others who have exemplified not only generosity but also the power and dignity that goes with being able to give a gift. Since the ultimate rationale for the conventional taboo against accepting gifts is to be sure that clients are talking freely rather than acting out their thoughts and feelings, it expresses a dangerous confusion of means and ends for a therapist to implement the "rule" of nonacceptance of gifts in instances where the appreciation of a gift will facilitate the client's self-disclosure, and the rejection of it will most likely provoke an injured withdrawal (cf. Whitson, 1996).

A myth exists—and persists with astonishing stubbornness—that people who are poor, marginal, alienated from the dominant culture, or unconventional in some important way are not good candidates for analytically oriented therapy. While it is true that people in such groups usually require some education as to what the therapy process is all about, and also require a special sensitivity and flexibility based on the therapist's appreciation of their special circumstances, there is no evidence that the verbal, insight-oriented therapies are not adaptable for people in such populations. In fact, it may represent one of the most arrogant forms of prejudice for people in the dominant sectors of a culture to pronounce its minority members "unsuited" to the collaborative, verbal, in-depth therapies (cf. Singer, 1970; Javier, 1990; Altman, 1995; Thompson, 1996). But it is true that therapists who work with people significantly different from themselves in terms of ethnicity, religion, race, class, culture, and sexual orientation have some extra work to do in their efforts to understand both the identifications of those they treat and their own silent prejudices and assumptions.

SUMMARY

In this chapter, I have explored the significance and treatment implications of a patient's individual identifications. I have commented on the developmental range of internalization processes—from primitive introjective phenomena to subjectively voluntary and nuanced identifications—and described how the nature and developmental tone of someone's internalized objects can be deduced from his or her transference reactions. I have explored some clinical implications of understanding both identifications and counteridentifications, and I have concluded with some observations about the clinical importance of appreciating the contributions of ethnicity, race, religion, class, culture, and minority status to anyone's psychology.

CHAPTER EIGHT

Assessing Relational Patterns

C LOSELY related to the question of a person's identifications is that of his or her repetitive ways of relating to other people. Where the issue of identification addresses mainly *who* are the patient's models, and *what* were the qualities about them that he or she wants to assimilate or reject, the issue of relational pattern concerns *how* the person's connections with his or her main love objects were expressed. A mother can be loving and positively valued, and her daughter may want to be like her in many ways, yet the primary way the girl has learned to relate to her may be compliant or rebellious, withdrawn or involved, demanding or self-abnegating, or any one of a virtually limitless number of possibilities. The interpersonal styles of caregivers and the underlying themes about relationship that they express are taken in by children, along with the more static qualities that people tend to refer to as "traits." In Chapter Seven I discussed internalized objects; in this one, I discuss the more complex topic of internalized object relations.

Specific questions about relationship patterns are often unnecessary in an intake interview. Because recurring interpersonal problems are among the chief reasons people seek psychotherapy, clients will frequently begin the session with a description of a persistent, maladaptive pattern of relationship. "I keep falling in love with abusive men," or "Every time I get excited about someone, I find her flaws and get disillusioned," or "I have this problem with authorities" are common responses to the therapist's opening invitation to patients to describe what brings them to a mental health professional. When a relational pattern is the chief complaint, one's formulation about it can be comparatively straightforward. When the presenting problem is a mood disturbance or obsessional thought or posttraumatic reaction or something else not conspicuously embedded in an interpersonal theme, the therapist must infer the central relational conflicts from transference data and historical information. Sometime it is also helpful to ask questions such as, "How would you describe your most important relationships?" or "What is your marriage like?" or "Are you close to anyone?" or "What do you value in people?" But the most reliable information tends to appear in the client's responses to the therapist.

Let me begin with a couple of examples of recurrent relational patterns that can show themselves in the first meeting of treatment. I recently interviewed a woman who wanted to see me for therapy. She explained that she had a persistent tendency to idealize male authorities and, despite a happy marriage, to become infatuated with certain men. I listened, felt warmly disposed toward her, felt I could probably help her with her problem, and found myself looking forward to working with her. Toward the end of our meeting, when she was recounting her prior experiences in therapy and counseling—all with female practitioners—I asked whether she had ever thought about going to a male therapist, given that her repetitive patterns with men might be immediately stimulated in such a situation. Her face fell, and I could tell that she interpreted my question as meaning that I did not want to work with her.

She very quickly started considering that it might be a good idea to see a man. She began to ask me about male practitioners in the area, but it was clear that her heart was not in this conversation. When I stopped her and explained that I had only been curious, that I had simply wanted to find out her thinking about having chosen only female therapists, she still looked skeptical. She seemed to feel driven to take care of me rather than to stand for her own needs and decisions, and if I wanted to get rid of her, she was not going to give me trouble. As we investigated this, we found a whole recurrent pattern of compliance and caretaking, secondary to fears of rejection, that characterized her behavior with both women and men.

Another person I recently interviewed with the objective of finding a referral for her, because I did not have room in my practice for a new patient, was a deeply dysthymic woman. She speculated that the source of her depression was a family history in which she had been the last child, an unplanned one, and that she had always felt treated like excess baggage. Her parents were overburdened, financially strapped, and preoccupied during her early years, and she never had the feeling that they were interested in listening to her. She commented that she had learned to keep her private feelings very carefully hidden from them. She had had several previous therapies, but she thought they had only made her feel guiltier about how little energy she had. I felt at the end of the interview that my understanding of her was disturbingly incomplete.

With her permission, I called the social worker who had referred her to me for evaluation and asked her perceptions about what kind of practitioner would be a good match for this woman. To my surprise, she told me that to her way of thinking, this client had never had real psychotherapy. She had been to a succession of people who called themselves Christian counselors and mainly used persuasion and Biblical authority to tell patients how they should be feeling and behaving. She had decided she would go to a more conventionally trained therapist, but she was nervous about it, because she was a deeply religious woman who expected a secular practitioner to debunk her faith. In fascinating parallel to the secretive way she had survived her mother's lack of availability to her (probably reinforced by my literal unavailability to take her on as a regular patient), she had not told me any of this.

A therapist needs to become familiar with the internal world of a client. Are its inhabitants generous or stingy, controlling or permissive, impinging or distancing, validating or undermining, exploitive or supportive, autocratic or consensual, merciful or punitive, critical or accepting, warm or cold, active or passive, inhibited or expressive, passionate or indifferent, involved or negligent, predictable or chaotic, stoic or self-indulgent? What were the patient's reactions to the childhood emotional environment? What repetitive conflicts occurred? The subtleties of a person's interpersonal history live on in current relationships, color the therapeutic connection, and constitute an area the clinician must address if he or she is to wield any therapeutic influence.

This observation has been made, with some variation in emphasis and yet with extraordinary commonality of overall conceptualization, by a remarkably diverse group of researchers. Some of them have influenced each other; others have started from isolated positions or less mainstream theoretical assumptions and have found that their data led them to similar relational phenomena. I am thinking of concepts such as Malan's (1976) "nuclear conflict," Gill and Hoffman's (1982) "patient's experience of the relationship with the therapist," Bucci's (1985) "referential set," Stern's (1985) "Representations of Interactions that have been Generalized" ("RIGs"), Henry, Schacht, and Strupp's (1986) "cyclical maladaptive pattern," Tomkins's "nuclear scene" (see Carlson, 1986), Weiss, Sampson, and colleagues' (1986) "higher mental functioning hypothesis," Dahl's (1988) "fundamental repetitive and maladaptive emotional structure" or "frames," Horowitz's (1988) "personal schema," the "model scenes" concept of Lachmann and Lichtenberg (1992), the "core conflictual relationship theme" of Luborsky and Crits-Christoph (1998), and Bretherton's (1998) concept of "representations." Lorna Smith Benjamin's (1993) empirically derived Structural Analysis of Social Behavior represents one of the most thoroughgoing empirical research projects whose outcome is consistent with this emphasis on the patterning of relationship as crucially diagnostic. In some nonpsychoanalytic writing, one finds a similar emphasis on repetitive patterns, for example, in the work of Klerman and his colleagues (Klerman, Weissman, Rounsaville, & Chevron, 1984) on "interpersonal psychotherapy."

Long before researchers identified repetitive scripts (templates, story lines, cognitive maps, personal tapes, subjective constructions—pick your metaphor) as central to an understanding of individual psychology and psychopathology, therapists were impressed with the recurrent nature of a limited number of themes in their clients' internal worlds and external relationships. Immersion in the effort to help people hour after hour puts a practitioner repeatedly in a role that elicits each patient's unique set of assumptions about authority, dependency, intimacy, gender, power, emotion, and other aspects of relationship. The contemporary psychodynamic clinical literature usually refers to recurring interpersonal configurations as "internalized object relations" (e.g., Kernberg, 1976; Ogden, 1986; Bollas, 1987; Horner, 1991; Scharff & Scharff, 1987, 1992). Sandler and Rosenblatt's (1962) concept of the individual's subjective "representational world" and Atwood and Stolorow's (1984) emphasis on "structures of subjectivity" are related concepts in that they are attempts to capture this dimension of individual psychology. A popularized and highly simplified approach to understanding relational themes appeared in the 1970s in Eric Berne's (1974) "transactional analysis," with its portrayal of certain common "games" or "scripts."

In psychotherapy, the issues that get hashed and rehashed ("worked through") between the patient and therapist, and between the patient and the main people in his or her life, tend to be repetitive dramas that after a while are excruciatingly familiar to both client and clinician. If Oliver Wendell Holmes was right that we all have one speech to give, and we give it repeatedly in various forms all our lives, it is also true that every person in therapy seems to have one main relational territory to explore and expand on, no matter how many different directions there are from which to approach that area. We all have our repetitive patterns, many of which are adaptive and benign. We come to psychotherapists when our central theme is problematic because it embodies a persistent and unremitting conflict. For example, we long for closeness but behave in ways that distance people, or we seek release from inhibition but fear our impulsivity, or we desire autonomy but feel shame and doubt when we act from a position of agency.

RELATIONAL THEMES IN THE TRANSFERENCE

The phenomenon of transference has sometimes been misunderstood as a straightforward displacement of childhood attitudes toward caregivers. It is actually much more complex. Whole atmospheres and intensities and defensive constellations get transferred into the clinical situation. The therapist cannot be limited to the questions that Freud identified as most important—namely, "Who am I to this person?" and "Is that figure mainly positive or mainly negative?" He or she must also feel out the nuances and meanings of what is transferred. There is a two-step process in this aspect of assessment: (1) How can one describe the pattern that keeps being reenacted? and (2) What are the origins, meanings, motives, and reinforcers of that pattern for this person?

Let me illustrate via attention to a fairly common pattern: the tendency to sexualize relationships. This proclivity may become evident as early as during an initial interview; for example, when a heterosexual female patient is in treatment with a male therapist. Parenthetically, let me comment that most therapists concur that a sexualizing tendency is not as immediate and observable when the patient is a heterosexual male in treatment with a female therapist, probably because in Western cultures the combination of higher-authority female with lower-authority male is not perceived as having the same erotic potential. Such a pattern is also likely to take a while to appear in the transference when the patient is gay or lesbian and of the same gender as the therapist, especially if the therapist is assumed to be heterosexual, probably because of the client's inhibition of yearnings that are socially disparaged.

Popular impressions aside, the phenomenon of "falling in love with one's analyst" is neither inevitable nor easily comprehended. Freud was the first person to try to make sense of such reactions, and he oversimplified them greatly. He saw erotic transferences as representing the displacement of positive sexual strivings from infantile objects to current ones. In other words, he would understand a heterosexual woman who became sexually preoccupied with her male therapist as reexperiencing feelings she once consciously had toward her father, feelings that had been repressed at the end of her oedipal period. Analysts have long known that an erotic transference represents much more than this; sexualization or erotization of a therapeutic relationship is never uncomplicated. (Some kinds of love in psychotherapy, in contrast, are quite straightforward and not highly conflicted. As Bergmann, 1987, has noted, the experience of coming to love a therapist is an expectable and therapeutically essential aspect of the treatment process. In fact, analytic psychotherapy derives its effectiveness from just such feelings. The more emotionally important a therapist is to a client, the more power he or she has to counteract the negative effects of the passionately loved and tenaciously internalized early caregivers.)

Contemporary therapists are open to many alternative possibilities in understanding a person's erotization of the therapy relationship. I do not refer to passing erotic feelings here, which occur in all relationships, including professional ones, but a chronic immersion in fantasies of being the therapist's lover. For example, the client's persistent sexual attraction to the therapist can indicate an identification with a powerful and seductive mother. Or it can be based on the opposite attitude, embodying the unconscious conviction that power is a male prerogative and that men must therefore be seduced into sharing it. Or it may be an attempt to master by passive-into-active transformation (Weiss et al., 1986) the anxieties created by childhood molestation. Or it may contain a wish to defeat a hated parent by luring the therapist out of his professional role. Sexualization with a man may be the way a woman learned as an emotionally deprived girl to satisfy her needs for nurturance and warmth. Or it may betray a defensive need to prove that she is not a lesbian. Or it may express a deeply valued victory over erotic inhibition. Or it may represent a general pattern of being unable to feel sexual with anyone other than forbidden figures. Or it may be a woman's desperate attempt to bring life and feeling to a situation that otherwise feels annihilating and dead. A persistently sexualized transference can be a manifestation of any of these dynamics, and many others, and will usually turn out to be a combination of several different unconscious attitudes that have overdetermined an erotic stance (see Gabbard, 1994, 1996).

The empirical literature on the disturbing frequency of sexual misuse of patients by therapists (Pope, 1989) and the analytic literature on boundary violations (Gabbard & Lester, 1995) attest to a problem of considerable magnitude. Its existence suggests that the complex possible meanings of a patient's erotization are not well understood by many practitioners, who apparently prefer to see their clients' attractions to them as expectable reactions to their intrinsic desirability. But even setting aside the problem of disastrous sexual enactments fueled by therapists' narcissism, clinicians must figure out how to free their individual patients of sexual preoccupations so that they can make use of treatment to resolve the problems they came in to address. The erotization of a therapeutic relationship calls for more than ethical clarity and routine tact. Whether one addresses the phenomenon by interpretation, confrontation, limit setting, or quiet tolerance of an important striving that will eventually run its course depends on one's appreciating the main relational meaning to a particular person of an erotized connection.

A client's tendency to approach connection with another person in a certain way will manifest itself in an initial interview and must be factored into an overall formulation. Accuracy in formulating a case depends partly on a practitioner's ability to use his or her subjectivity to understand the probable meaning of a relational form that is being sculpted by a patient. In addition to reflecting on information from the person's history that might explain the centrality of some specific relational tendency, a sensitive therapist uses his or her internal emotional responses diagnostically. To illustrate how one does this, let me continue with the example of a person who tends to sexualize relationships. One's subjective reaction to a seductive patient can be dominated, among other possibilities, by enjoyment, fear, irritation, sexual excitement, or narcissistic inflation. Each reaction would be saying something different about what erotization does for this particular patient.

Naturally, because interviewers' reactions will be a combination of their own relational proclivities and the emotional forces that are making an impact on them, well-trained therapists try to sort out what is "theirs" from what the client brings to the interaction (Roland, 1981). In fact, many contemporary psychoanalysts emphasize the "co-construction" of the transference (e.g., Orange, 1995) by the subjectivities of both participants in the therapy process. One reason for the stress that psychoanalytic training institutes have traditionally placed on the personal analysis of the therapist is that awareness of one's own patterns allows one to distinguish between what a client is inducing and what the therapist is inclined to feel in any interpersonal situation.

Over the years, I have concluded that many analytic supervisors overemphasize the need for beginning therapists to identify their "own stuff" when a client stirs them up. If this is the main direction one takes when a patient activates some affective potential, one can get lost in self-analysis and may conclude that the resolution of a difficult affective state between two people is going to depend mainly on the therapist's working through his or her own conflicts. This is a misguided notion, both because perfect self-knowledge and self-control are unattainable and because patients come to resolve their own conflicts, not those of their therapists. More to the point, such a focus distracts practitioners from attending to the emotional forces that are acting on them, thus depriving both parties of a deeper understanding of what the patient is bringing to the interaction. However significant the therapist's emotional contribution to what goes on between the parties to the therapeutic dyad, for diagnostic purposes, it is important first to get a sense of what the patient seems to bring to any interaction.

Having made that point, I should add the caveat that just feeling something in the presence of a client does not automatically mean that the client is "putting" that feeling there. The appreciation of the diagnostic value of countertransference reactions, a liberative position that at this point is comfortably mainstream, has unfortunately contributed to a glib tendency in some practitioners to ascribe automatically to patients whatever uncomfortable states of mind they notice in themselves (e.g., "I'm feeling angry now, so you must be trying to make me angry" or "I feel confused, so that must be how you *really* feel"). Knowing that the therapist's subjectivity may say a lot about the client's does not obviate the need for discipline, introspection, and the weighing of more than one explanatory possibility.

Many years ago, I conducted an intake interview with a man who immediately called me "Nance," held the office door for me, and complimented me on my outfit. He seemed to need to relate to me entirely in a flirtation mode. I felt irritated by his manner and noted in myself an inclination to get prissy and judgmental with him, as if to say, "Your behavior is very inappropriate in a professional situation." Not wanting to act out that response to his seductiveness before I understood it, I tried to remain warm while boundaried, and I proceeded to collect information on his personal history. It turned out that he had experienced his mother as extremely dominating and even sadistic in her treatment of him. I began to see that one function of his flirtatiousness was an effort to express dominance over women he saw as potentially powerful. My irritation was expressing my defensive reaction to his effort to put me in a one-down position. Intriguingly, later in the hour, when I commented nonjudgmentally on his tendency to flirt with me, his reaction was to feel exposed and bereft of an important "weapon." He then proceeded to get too sleepy to attend to the rest of the interview. He somewhat reluctantly went on to describe a recurring pattern with women who interested him (and it was only relatively powerful women who did): He would try first to dazzle them. If that failed to work, he would become unbearably weary in their presence. I took this man into treatment, but he and I soon decided that this dynamic was too oppressive for our particular therapeutic partnership—it is not easy do therapy with someone who keeps falling asleep—and I referred him on to a man with whom he did well, because they could talk about his pattern with women without having it immediately sabotage their sessions.

Another man I worked with for many years contributed more subtly and slowly to an erotic feeling between us. As I found myself preoccupied with sexual fantasies during his hour, I felt a disturbing combination of both sexual excitement and fear. I also felt a strong wish to ignore these feelings, to behave with him as if there were nothing erotic in the atmosphere, and certainly nothing that was turning me on. After a while, I felt so disingenuous working with him without commenting on the "vibes" I kept feeling that I brought up my sense that there was some sexual material that he and I seemed to be complicit in avoiding (cf. Davies, 1994). He responded first with denial and then with fear and shame. Although he had not told me in the initial interview that he had ever suffered sexual abuse, he had powerful associations to a repetitive experience with his mother, who gave him enemas in a ritualized, sadistic, and erotized way from the time he was three to the time he was seven. He felt both traumatized and excited by this special, secret activity that she imposed on him regularly. Outside the drama of the enemas, they had a tacit compact never to mention their clandestine rituals. My excitement, fear, and wish to disregard the sexual atmosphere mirrored this complex interpersonal dynamic, which later became obvious as a problem in many of his relationships.

Another client who created a sexual atmosphere in my office induced in me a radically different emotional reaction. He was a profoundly inhibited, schizoid man who had sought treatment at thirty-six, when he began to feel there was something wrong with his remaining single and virginal despite numerous opportunities to develop serious relationships with women, many of whom he was ravishing in his private fantasy life. His psychology was dominated by a counteridentification with a father who had been a guiltless philanderer, and who pressed him from his early teens to join him in seeking the services of prostitutes. In his mind, sex was all bound up with submission to his father's perverse agenda, which included a thinly disguised compulsion to demean women. My client loved his mother and refused to play this game.

In response to my invitation toward the end of the interview to comment on his reaction to me, this patient mentioned that he found me attractive. My subjective response in this case was simply pleasure—not only the narcissistic inflation that is a natural reaction to being complimented but also a more maternal kind of anticipation of his possible capacity to feel and name an erotic inclination that was different from his father's driven sexualizing. Unlike many erotic transferences, his mental erotization of the therapy relationship turned out not to be primarily a resistance to other material (like power issues or memories of an abuse history, as in the two previous examples). Instead, it represented the emergence of a potential for growth toward intimacy that eventually expressed itself in a sexual relationship with a woman he had liked and admired for years. My initial countertransference had been benign at least partly because in this man, there was a benign developmental process going on rather than a more conflicted, resistive one (cf. Trop, 1988).

I have used sexualized interactions to illustrate the phenomena I want to discuss in this section partly because they are among the most difficult for therapists to deal with, and partly because I find that contemporary students of therapy are hesitant to acknowledge and explore their more sexual reactions to clients. (Perhaps our training programs have put so much emphasis on discouraging sexual enactments that therapists fear even to notice any evidence of arousal.) But the same principles apply to the appearance in the transference of any interpersonal dynamic and all its emotional trappings. A therapist who is fully open to the feelings that a client stirs up—even upsetting ones such as sexual arousal, hatred, sadism, shame, boredom, contempt, and envy—will find that a whole drama (a "family romance" in the evocative language of Freud) will unfold in the therapy room and consequently open itself up to new plot twists, characters, and resolutions via the therapy process.

Respective Implications of Transference Themes in Psychoanalysis and in Psychotherapy

In classical psychoanalytic treatment, the gradual re-creation between the analyst and analysand of the core conflictual relationship has been called the *transference neurosis* (Freud, 1920). People who have quipped that psychoanalysis creates an illness in order to cure it are not entirely wrong: The analytic situation encourages problematic relational patterns to emerge in exquisite detail and in full emotional intensity. The mutual identification and then working through of a transference neurosis are, in fact, the qualitative features that differentiate psychoanalysis proper from less ambitious treatments. The technical procedures that maximize the chances for a transference neurosis to become manifest (use of the couch, free association, high frequency of sessions, unlimited time) are often cited as definitional of analysis as opposed to analytically oriented therapy, but in fact, they are only the conditions under which a full analysis is likely to become possible. (It is well known that, among healthier people who are motivated for analytic work, some can experience the flowering and pruning of a transference neurosis in twice-per-week treatment, while others in five-times-per-week analysis fail to experience the full replication of the core relational pattern in the analytic partnership. So far, despite lavish attention to the question of "analyzability," no one has yet figured out how one can reliably tell one kind of client from the other at the outset of treatment [Greenson, 1967; Etchegoyen, 1991].) It is this controlled but regressive experience of being reimmersed in early emotional relationships that allows the therapist and patient together to appreciate the power of an individual's interpersonal themes and repetitions, to understand in depth why they have so much power, and to develop new ways of resolving the conflicts they contain.

Classical analysis is widely considered to be the treatment of choice for people with high ego strength, high motivation, and professional or personal interest in going as deeply as possible into their personal subjective world. It is not the best treatment for people in the borderline or psychotic ranges of character structure, or for people with certain kinds of pathology (e.g., dissociative symptoms, paranoid tendencies) even if they are in the neurotic range. And there are many circumstances in which, even if it were the ideal approach, it is not practical. In less intensive therapies, treater and client work with transference reactions rather than a fully elaborated transference neurosis, but the aims are the same: to feel out the recurring conflicts as they appear in the treatment and then to devise together a different set of resolutions for them.

Psychodynamic therapy is harder to do than classical psychoanalysis. In analysis, relational patterns emerge gradually and naturally, relatively uncontaminated by the therapist's pressure to focus on what he or she considers the main interpersonal issues. Practitioners working at a lesser frequency, or in time-limited situations, or with patients for whom analysis would stimulate too much uncontrolled regression, must be more attentive to formulating dynamics before they are painfully obvious. They must be more active in their interventions and more willing to risk being off base or outright wrong about the patterns they begin to discern. Despite some residues of prejudice to the effect that analysis is inherently superior to dynamically oriented therapy (a prejudice that has supported the narcissism of psychoanalysts but seems to have been only obliquely related to clinical outcomes [Wallerstein, 1986]), contemporary clinicians seem to be appreciating that more limited therapies—including expressive and supportive treatments—are harder to conduct, require more creativity, and often meet a patient's needs more adequately than analysis proper.

Relational Patterns Conspicuously Absent from the Transference

Conscientious therapists not only feel out the nature of relationships that repeat themselves in the therapeutic dyad, but they also sense what kinds of relating are absent in a client's experience. This is a more difficult aspect of diagnosis than articulating what relational paradigms are present, for it requires an empathic leap into areas of void and lack that the patient by definition cannot verbalize. A malnourished person brought up entirely on gruel may know that something is wrong, but he or she has no concept of salad. An important aspect of formulating a case is the assessment of what kinds of relating have never been part of a person's experience, and then figuring out how to introduce such concepts in an emotionally salient way so that the patient may mourn what he or she missed and acquire capacities that he or she could not have previously imagined. The empathic leap into what is missing, not just what is present and problematic, did not characterize most general clinical theory until fairly recently, when *deficit* formulations such as those of the self psychologists and intersubjectivists (e.g., Kohut, 1977; Stolorow & Lachmann, 1980; Ornstein & Ornstein, 1985; Stolorow, Brandschaft, & Atwood, 1987; Wolf, 1988) were developed. Since their contributions, therapists have had more models for understanding previously unemphasized aspects of their patients' emotional needs and predicaments.

I have long suspected that the etiological speculations of the 1950s and 1960s attributing numerous psychopathologies to maternal failings were products of a clinical situation that mirrored the cultural child-rearing climate of too much mother and not enough father. In other words, people whose fathers had been conspicuous by their emotional absence tended to bring internalized mother issues into the treatment room. Patients knew they were upset with their mothers; they often did not know that if they had had more of a father on the scene, mother would not have looked so bad or loomed so large. They might not have had to put so much energy into getting out from under her. It was less painful, and more concrete, to lament a mother's sins of commission than a father's sins of omission. Therapists also found it more compelling to deal with what was being transferred—that is, they were repetitively seen as Mother because they were there and involved—than with what was absent from the transference, namely, a paternal dimension of experience.

It is just as important to assess what relational patterns are *not* evident in a client's style of connecting with a therapist as it is to feel fully the ones that are. Once, during an early session with a man who had come to me in a depression that he connected to having turned thirty-nine, I noticed that he tended to reiterate things he had already told me. "I get the feeling you weren't always listened to very carefully," I commented. "What do you mean, 'listened to'?" he asked, with an edge of sarcasm on the word *listened*. "I don't know exactly," I answered, "but you tend to repeat things to me as if I don't pay much attention to what you say. I thought maybe some of the people who brought you up had been distracted or preoccupied, and that you had gotten used to reminding them of what you had previously said." His response was, "Do you mean that most parents *listen* to their children?" This was a novel concept to him. Everyone takes his or her family of origin as modal, and often it is quite late in adulthood that one can identify what was missing and never consciously missed in that family.

Contemporary scholars in trauma and dissociation (e.g., McFarlane & van der Kolk, 1996) are currently stressing something similar. Despite the fact that what captures one's attention with people who have traumatic early histories—of sexual abuse or physical maltreatment or painful medical invasions, for example—one of the most important things to understand about their psychologies is the role of neglect. What was not there in their young lives is just as important as what was. Almost any experience can be rendered nontraumatic if someone spends sufficient time with a child to help him or her understand and emotionally process what happened. At least after the age of two, when children can verbalize, it is often not so much the trauma itself that is pathogenic, but rather the atmosphere of minimization and denial with which a family treats it. When one interviews an abuse victim, the description of the horrors inflicted on him or her may be riveting. But a therapist should also take note of what is absent from the drama that has been reported: No one listened to the abused youngster, offered comfort, helped the child verbalize what happened, modeled a way of coping. These will be the more therapeutic aspects of the subsequent relationship with a clinician.

RELATIONAL THEMES OUTSIDE THE THERAPY SITUATION

Not everything is discernible in the transference, by its presence or its absence, especially in an intake session. One important reason for taking a detailed look into a prospective client's past—taking family, social, sexual, work, and prior therapy histories—is to discern patterns of relationship that repeat in different forms over the years and across situations. An appreciation of recurrent themes can have value not only in suggesting the emphases that will eventually be therapeutic to an individual client, but also for solidifying enough of a working alliance to keep that person coming back.

Of particular importance in this area is attaining a description of other therapies the client has had, especially in those people who have made several previous, failed attempts to resolve their problems with other professionals. Notwithstanding the possibility that a candidate for therapy has had the bad luck to run into several badly trained or untalented practitioners, the best preliminary hypothesis for an interviewer to make is that what happened to the previous therapists will happen to oneself. Sorting out exactly what the client's complaints are about prior treatment is critical for two reasons. First, if one understands them well enough, one may be able to avoid some of the mistakes made by one's predecessors. For example, identifying how previous treaters may have become involved in some problematic enactment can give one advance notice on how to prepare for handling that situation. Second, and more important, since it is more than likely that one will be "caught," despite one's preparations, in the same mistakes other professionals have made (if not objectively, at least from the client's perspective), a careful examination of the pattern of prior therapeutic failure gives one the opportunity to predict to the client that the same thing may very well happen in this therapy. Could he or she manage not to flee treatment this time but instead verbalize the anger and disappointment?

When I learn from a patient that he or she has seen a bevy of prior therapists, that no one has really understood this suffering person before, that I am the last hope, my vanity is instantly activated. I find myself eager to assure such clients that, unlike the professionals they have seen before me, I can help them. Years of practice have humbled me— not enough to have changed this internal reaction, but enough to avoid acting it out. I now explicitly take the position that I will make mistakes, that they will probably be similar in some way to the mistakes that others have made, and that the client and I can use these failures of mine to understand together something important and find a constructive way to react. This communication rescues both the patient and me from unrealistic demands and conveys the message that when people disappoint, something other than despair may come out of the experience.

Early in my career as a therapist, I became interested in working with people of a psychopathic inclination. I liked expanding my therapeutic repertoire to embrace the difference in style that such patients seemed to require—namely, a more hard-nosed, tough-talking, tell-it-like-it-is confrontational tone so dramatically unlike the softer, more manifestly sympathetic approach that touches most other patients. I felt critical of the naivete of other therapists who had failed to help such clients. I had been taught that it was very important not to let an antisocial client "get over" on the therapist, and I tried to call such clients on every manipulation they attempted, lest I be seen as a "mark" and immediately devalued (see Bursten, 1973). This is fine as far as it goes, but I soon learned that no matter how clever I was, a psychopathic client could find a way to succeed in manipulating me. So I concluded that the most important therapeutic communication is not "Just try—you're not going to be able to con me," but rather "Listen, you can certainly con me if that's what you insist on doing during your appointments—I have no magical way of distinguishing between the truth and a convincing lie—but is that really how you want to spend your time here?" Competition with prior therapists or with imagined other practitioners who lack one's special skills is fine as an internal state, but it can be disastrous if acted out.

Interpersonal patterns that emerge from taking a social, sexual, and work history may also predict problems in treatment and suggest preemptive action. An apposite instance would be the person who reports leaving relationships (friends, jobs, or sexual partners) whenever they begin to seem constricting, or when the person begins to feel exposed, or when he or she notices a feeling of deep attachment or dependency.

This kind of pattern is not only fraught with the loneliest kind of suffering—on the part of both the patient and the people left behind—but is also one of the problems for which analytic therapy can be most profoundly healing. That is, if the person can be kept in treatment. When someone reports what sounds like extreme, automatic, and compulsive retreat from relationship whenever he or she gets too connected, it behooves a therapist to make an immediate contract with the client not to act that response out unreflectively. Specifically, the two parties make a pact that if the pattern of fleeing appears in treatment—if the person abruptly decides, whatever the reason (money and time are the most common ones), to terminate precipitously—the client will come back for a designated number of sessions to process what has happened. This precaution has saved more than one treatment of which I have personal knowledge. In instances where the person decided to leave anyway, at least he or she had the experience of talking rather than just acting under emotional duress, and conceivably learned something important in the process. With luck, the next therapist will benefit from the client's expanded self-knowledge.

Sexual patterns contain relational themes in a highly charged, condensed form. Clinical experience suggests that repetitive sexual motifs express either the dominant interpersonal patterns in an individual's life or a sequestered, partially dissociated relationship theme that appears only in sex and needs to be integrated into the person's larger experiential world. If an interviewer can speak with ease about sexuality, a client often reacts with relief that his or her private and possibly shame-filled erotic life is not so mysterious or kinky that it defies articulation. A clinician's candor and comfort about sex encourages frank disclosure and promotes hope in clients that the difficulties in their love lives can be ameliorated. Therapists who have trouble talking explicitly should practice naming sexual activities and body parts aloud to trusted friends. Some of my supervision groups have spent a meeting doing this; members generally experience a combination of excitement, discomfort, embarrassment, and hilarity, but the exercise contributes to a verbal disinhibition that is essential for therapists.

The directive to be forthright applies with special urgency to the interviewing of lesbian, gay, bisexual, and transgendered people, as well as those with presenting sexual problems such as paraphilias and compulsive enactments ("sex addiction," in the trendy language of recent years). Minimally, such patients need to know that a mental health professional will not be shocked by their sexual predilections; ideally, they should feel that their interviewer has a genuine appreciation of and respect for erotic diversity. With gay patients, for example, queries such as, "Are your sexual preferences more oral or more anal?" and "Do you tend to be a 'bottom' or a 'top'?" can cast light on important relational issues. With bisexual people, investigation of the differing gratifications they experience with women and men, respectively, can be illuminating. The more frank a therapist's tone, the better, although when one treads on delicate personal ground, it is considerate to tell clients that they are free not to answer any questions that feel too intrusive. It is also important to reflect a client's choice of sexual terms; for example, if a man refers to "coming," the interviewer should not then refer to his "ejaculating."

Because all kinds of human motives can be sexualized, the knowledge of a person's particular sexual pattern reveals something about his or her primary preoccupations. Some people sexualize their dependency (valuing the oral and cuddling aspects of sex to the exclusion of other factors); others sexualize their aggression (prizing the dominance and submission aspects); still others use sex mostly in the service of narcissistic needs (valuing the exhibitionistic and voyeuristic features of sexuality, or the illusion of having one's desires magically known and wordlessly satisfied, or the fantasy of defeating and humiliating the other party). Sometimes, especially when there is a childhood history of physical suffering connected with the genitals (from sexual abuse, accidents, or medical procedures), the enduring or inflicting of pain may be a prerequisite to orgasm. In any of these circumstances, a relational theme is embodied starkly in the sexual domain.

IMPLICATIONS OF RELATIONAL PATTERNS FOR LONG-TERM VERSUS SHORT-TERM THERAPIES

In open-ended therapies, except for instances in which flight from treatment is an obvious risk, one can confidently expect core relational themes to emerge over time. An interviewer who misses some central interpersonal motif in the initial interview has not usually committed a grave oversight, because any theme of import will express itself with unmistakable clarity sooner or later. In time-limited therapies, however, the practitioner's capacity to zero in on the most central conflictual relational pattern is critical to making use of the short time at his or her disposal. For the reader unfamiliar with the empirical literature on short-term dynamic therapy, I recommend the work of my colleagues Stanley Messer and Seth Warren (1995), who note the recurrence of this emphasis on understanding a patient's central relational dynamics in most of the current major approaches to time-limited analytic treatment.

In longer-term therapies and in psychoanalysis proper, one of the motives for change that I have rarely seen discussed in the analytic literature is the fact that patients ultimately get self-conscious, chagrined, and even bored hearing themselves describe the same interactions over and over again. After a while, it becomes easier to try something new than to go back to one's therapist and confess that one has once more acted out the same old pattern. Naming and describing one's central "neurosis" *ad nauseam* in the presence of a witness to one's irrationality, leading to eventual feelings of ennui and exasperation in both parties, make the risk of new behavior feel better than the misery of repetition. This motivational benefit is probably one of the great unresearched contributants to change in psychotherapy. But it can only happen if the therapist has identified a pattern, named it, and created a safe environment where it can be talked about again and again. Thus, the sooner one can capture a relational dynamic in words, the faster one can help a person to change it into some healthier way of dealing with other people.

SUMMARY

In this chapter, I have discussed how and why one attempts to understand the repetitive interpersonal themes that dominate the subjective life of an individual patient. I have emphasized that these patterns consist of dramas and conflicts, and therefore are appropriately understood as internalized object *relations,* not just internalized objects. I have referred to the empirical and clinical literatures on recurrent patterns of interaction and have explored how they manifest themselves both within and outside the treatment relationship. I have made some comparisons between psychoanalysis and psychotherapy, and between long- and short-term dynamic treatment, in terms of how such patterns become known to patient and practitioner and how they may be dealt with therapeutically.

I have tried to show how taking a good history can illuminate themes that will become central to treatment, themes that sometimes need to be understood and articulated immediately if the patient is to be kept from leaving the therapy relationship. With respect to relational patterns that appear in the therapeutic dyad, I have emphasized the diagnostic importance of the therapist's disciplined subjectivity. I have also stressed the value of noticing types of interpersonal relationship that are notable for their absence from a client's repertoire. Finally, I have mentioned briefly how a deep appreciation of the persistence of a central drama can support a person's motivation for change.

CHAPTER NINE

◁◖◉

Assessing Self-Esteem

SELF-ESTEEM, or what analysts sometimes call healthy narcissism, is another part of emotional life in which people differ strikingly. Anyone who wants to help others, in the short term or in a comprehensive way, needs to understand each client's individuality in this area. How secure is his or her self-esteem? On what is it based? What undermines it? How is it restored when it is injured? How realistic are the aspirations on which it depends? The specific conditions that support a person's self-regard constitute one of those taken-for-granted, unarticulated aspects of individual psychology, never fully conscious and always ego-syntonic, that operate like water to the fish. The means by which one feels good or bad about oneself is a fact of one's mental organization so pervasive, longstanding, and invisible that most of us cannot imagine handling our system of self-approval and disapproval any other way. Because self-esteem is a quintessentially internal phenomenon, its nature must be inferred from a client's behavior and verbal reports.

THE SIGNIFICANCE OF UNDERSTANDING
SELF-ESTEEM ISSUES

The preservation and enhancement of self-esteem is at the center of all mature human activity. People who find themselves acting in contradiction to their values will feel shame and despair to such an extent that they cannot be consoled. They will do things that put themselves or other people at risk rather than feel such anguish. They may accomplish things that most other people cannot imagine achieving. Freud, for example, has sometimes been gushingly idealized by psychoanalytic admirers who cannot fathom how anyone could have bulldozed through his own resistances and exposed his unconscious life to the extent that Freud did. But given his self-esteem structure, his accomplishment is not quite so incomprehensible. It was central to Freud's value system to see himself as fearless in his devotion to the truth, as a conquistador against hypocrisy and self-deception. He took great pleasure in uncovering in himself what to others would have been highly unpalatable aspects of their psychology. Whatever shame his discoveries cost him was amply counterbalanced by the infusion of pride he felt at buttressing his self-image as a dauntless truth-teller.

Cultures create shared values that make otherwise incomprehensible behaviors rather ordinary. For example, in contemporary American middle-class society, people whose self-esteem depends on looking young and beautiful will undergo extensive surgery rather than face the narcissistic suffering they associate with normal aging. In wartime, soldiers whose pride depends on acting bravely will face death rather than shame. As the *Titanic* was going down, Benjamin Guggenheim, raised with an Edwardian sensibility about what should matter to one's self-esteem, laid aside his lifebelt, and along with his secretary, changed into white tie and tails, declaring, "We've dressed in our best and are prepared to go down like gentlemen" (Butler, 1998, p. 123).

When I studied people who had spent their lives saving, healing, rescuing, and otherwise helping other people, often at considerable inconvenience or even physical risk to themselves (McWilliams, 1984), I learned that when they were prevented from doing their good deeds, they got depressed. A woman I know became significantly dysphoric after being diagnosed with breast cancer—not just because she feared for her life, but because her hospital would no longer allow her to donate blood regularly, an activity that was central to her feeling of value. Usually, when other people cannot understand a person's motivation for a given act, it is because they do not share, and cannot imagine sharing, that person's means of maintaining self-esteem. Therapists are used to hearing others ask them, "How can you stand it, sitting around all day listening to other people's troubles?" People who ask such questions probably do not have helping people at the center of their own value system; hence, they cannot imagine how the pleasure in helping can override the discomfort of absorbing intense negative affect hour after hour.

This lack of empathy for those whose self-esteem depends on different sources from one's own applies not only to heroic and "self-sacrificing" acts but also to destructive and evil ones. Someone whose self-regard is based on seeming independent and invulnerable can beat up a partner rather than express a need for that person; someone whose pride depends on feeling ultimate power over other people can prefer murder to the shame of inaction. Timothy McVeigh's destruction of the Oklahoma City Federal Building and so many of its innocent occupants was probably motivated not just by his famous hatred of the federal government but also by his sense that he could not maintain his self-esteem if he failed to act in accordance with his ideology. Such behavior is, of course, incomprehensible to people with contrasting ways of organizing their self-esteem.

In the absence of information about a particular person's self-esteem structure, we all tend to project, to assume that the things that make us feel good about ourselves are the same ones that instill pride in our clients. Self-esteem is intimately tied to the qualities we admire and idealize, in ourselves and others. But families and subcultures idealize remarkably different things, and it can be startling to appreciate how discrepantly self-esteem can be supported and maintained. One woman congratulates herself on her intellectuality, while another feels contempt for those with an "ivory tower mentality and no common sense." One man takes pains to be a fastidious dresser, while his neighbor nurses the conceit that physical appearance means nothing to him. A patient of mine who prided herself on her agnosticism spent a session expressing confusion and pain about the sexually restrained behavior of a man she was dating. She had concluded that he found her unattractive, yet except for his sexual conservatism, his behavior suggested the opposite. As she had previously mentioned that he had been raised Roman Catholic and still attended Mass regularly, I suggested an alternative explanation: "Perhaps he feels, in conformity with his religious upbringing, that premarital sex is wrong." "Surely nobody in this day and age can think *that*!" she exclaimed. But he did. And his self-esteem depended on his behaving accordingly. He was attracted to her, but he would not have been able to feel good about himself if he had engaged in sexual relations with her before marriage.

To learn about a patient's self-esteem, perhaps the most telling question to ask is, "What do you admire in people?" The answer supplies the main ingredient in the person's self-evaluation. It is also sometimes useful to ask specifically, "What kinds of things make you feel good about yourself?" and "What kinds of things get you down on yourself?" In addition, one may get a sense of the person's overall level of self-esteem by asking something like, "On balance, do you feel positive about yourself and your life, or are you disappointed and self-critical?" People who have trouble exposing their shame later in the therapy, once the therapist has become someone whose acceptance and admiration they seek, can often confess their worst feelings about themselves early in the treatment.

Here is perhaps a good place for me to comment on the difference between a sophisticated, psychoanalytic understanding of self-esteem and those that popular culture seems to have embraced, as evidenced in current arguments over issues such as grade inflation and social promotion. Praising and rewarding people for trivial accomplishments produces not self-esteem but self-deception and feelings of fraudulence. We react to cheap praise with either an inflated sense of ourselves that at some level we know is nonsense, or with the private shame that, notwithstanding the accolades, we are only mediocre. Typically, we also have disdain for the admirer. Children are notoriously more appreciative of demanding teachers than of lenient ones: They know that praise from someone with high standards means something.

"Supporting" people's self-esteem by giving them only positive reactions is not protecting or creating reasonable self-esteem; it is fostering illusion. If the recipient actually believes the praise, then he or she will set such low standards in the future that the possibility of feeling positive and successful in a complicated world will be obviated. One of the reasons that people's self-esteem improves during psychoanalysis is that, in contrast to the notion that authorities should reframe everything as good, the patient has exposed much that is bad and shameful, and the analyst has not shrunk from understanding those loathed parts of the self. The patient has been accepted by someone who knows all his or her faults, not someone who needs to minimize or distort. If superficial emotional support did anything substantial for a person's self-esteem, then anyone with friends would not need psychotherapy.

PSYCHOANALYTIC ATTENTION TO SELF-ESTEEM

Self-esteem did not reach center stage in the psychoanalytic tradition until about the 1970s, when there was a flood of writing and research on pathological narcissism—a condition defined by the inability to regulate self-esteem reasonably and consistently via internal standards of value. Therapists were finding that more and more of their clients were not describing problems of the traditional Freudian variety, in which their internal dynamics were in conflict, but instead were complaining of vague feelings of emptiness, meaninglessness, difficulty defining themselves, difficulty liking who they were, and envy of others presumed to "have it all" or "have it together." Sometimes these problems in feeling an internal center of gravity were overt; sometimes they were obscured by a grandiose self-presentation similar to what Wilhelm Reich (1933) had called "phallic narcissism." Certainly the kind of culture we now inhabit—with its chronic and dizzying change, international scope, mobility, emphasis on image and spin, and relative invisibility of any of us as individuals—makes it much harder to attain a stable sense of who we are and why we matter than was true in the kind of society that spawned the early psychoanalytic theorists.

Still, self-esteem difficulties are hardly the sole province of recent decades. Among analysts in Freud's early circle, both Adler (e.g., 1927), with his attention to problems reflecting the feeling of inferiority, and Rank (e.g., 1945), with his focus on the individual will, were writing about the self and the centrality of a stable self-esteem to people's well-being. Freud, whose personal dynamics were not marked by significant deficits in self-esteem, and who therefore probably lacked empathy for narcissistic problems, seems to have felt that emphases on self-esteem regulation were somewhat peripheral to an understanding of the neurotic conditions in which he was most interested.

The Psychoanalytic Focus on the Superego

Where classical psychoanalytic theory, notably in the ego psychology tradition, does touch on the issue of self-esteem is in the concept of the superego. In the Freudian model of development, children resolve their problematic sexual and aggressive urges by identification with their parents, especially the parent with whom they feel most competitive. The acceptance that "I can't possess Mommy, but I can have someone like Mommy if I become like Daddy" rescues a child from the condition of chronic, doomed longing and frustration. Becoming like a caregiver means internalizing that person's value system and making one's self-esteem contingent on behaving according to standards that one's parents or guiding authorities have set. In analytic writing before the debut of narcissism as a central preoccupation, there was considerable attention to how the superego arose, how it was influenced preoedipally, and whether it was reasonable or unduly harsh (e.g., Beres, 1958). Such articles were often inspired by the author's experience with depressive and obsessive–compulsive patients, whose notoriously demanding superegos made it very difficult for them to feel adequately positive about themselves.

Later, when borderline conditions excited widespread clinical interest, much attention was paid to the question of whether a person has an "integrated" superego. This label refers to the clinical observation that most people seem to have one overall, more or less reasonable set of values by which they judge themselves, an ethical compass that feels like a natural part of their personality. Their conscience and their moral aspirations are thus integrated with their consistent sense of who they are. A minority of clients seen in therapy, however, those who eventually became understood as having a borderline personality structure, bounce back and forth between feeling all-good and all-bad. They get into "ego states" (Kernberg, 1975) that are totalistic, that lack the sense of a tension between, for example, what one wants to do and what one's conscience decrees is permissible.

Most analysts presume that these clients get this way through a combination of individual temperament and childhood experience with caregivers who behaved in ways that made the oedipal phase too problematic to resolve by identification (love objects have to be reasonably idealizable in order to make the "traditional" oedipal resolution possible for a child). People with borderline personality organization thus vacillate between feeling that nothing they do could be wrong and feeling that everything they do is wrong. They lack an integrated sense that as long as they conform to reasonable moral standards, they are good enough. Naturally, a consistency in self-esteem is impossible for them, and they suffer greatly, often resorting to desperate measures to reinstate an internal sense of adequacy.

Our capacity to understand the kinds of problems posed by patients who are now understood to have borderline dynamics was significantly influenced by Erikson's (e.g., 1968) work on identity. So familiar have terms such as "identity crisis" become in popular lingo that one forgets that in the 1950s, when Erikson introduced the concept, it was a new idea. As I commented in Chapter One, identity is rarely a problem for people living in small, stable, intimate societies, where they and all their acquaintances know their defined role, but it becomes increasingly problematic in cultures like ours that are massive in scale, filled with conflicting messages, and demanding of constant change. In such a world, one cannot hang one's identity on a stable *role*: Current projections suggest that people who come of age at the millennium will change jobs an average of six times! Instead, one needs to feel a continuity of internal values and feelings that give the self a sense of solidity and reliability. As life became more complicated and imperiled during the twentieth century, psychoanalytic theory became more and more focused on how people maintain some sense of inner consistency and worth.

Humanistic and Existential Psychotherapy, Self Psychology, and the Intersubjectivists

Despite these areas of clinical observation and theory, traditional analytic writing in the middle decades of the twentieth century had certain lacunae in the area of understanding the sense of self and the vicissitudes of self-approval or its absence (see Menaker, 1995). Into that gap came the "third force" psychologists such as Carl Rogers, Abraham Maslow, and Gordon Allport, as well as the existential analysts such as Viktor Frankl and Rollo May. The great appeal of Rogerian psychotherapy, and of humanistic therapy in general at that time, may derive from Rogers's exquisite attunement to clients' self-esteem and to his appreciation of how fragile is the sense of self-worth of anyone seeking psychological help. Between the lines (e.g., Rogers, 1951), one can hear Rogers's outrage at the heavy-handed interpretive practices of many of the analytic psychiatrists of his day, who did not take into account how wounding their interventions could be to a vulnerable patient, even (perhaps especially) when the analyst was correct about the analysand's dynamics. Rogers's overarching emphasis on self-esteem, which influenced several generations of therapists of diverse theoretical orientations, probably laid the groundwork for an appreciation of Kohut and other analytic writers when they began to make similar observations in psychodynamic language.

The existentially oriented psychoanalysts, influenced greatly by the cataclysmic events of World War II and the Holocaust, emphasized at midcentury the sense of self and the problem of self-esteem for individuals. Viktor Frankl (1969) noted that the attributes that were conducive to good adaptation in the prewar world were not necessarily those that permitted personal transcendence of the horrors of existence in the concentration camps. Like the controversial Bruno Bettelheim, who also survived a wartime camp experience, he commented on the vast differences among people in their respective accommodations to extreme circumstances, noting that the capacity to sustain self-esteem had much more to do with psychical survival than did people's management of their sexuality and aggression.

All these influences, combining with Kohut's seminal work on narcissism and contemporaneous empirical researches into infancy and early childhood, produced a movement within psychoanalysis to redefine both developmental theory and clinical technique to reflect the central role of the self. One's sense of personal identity, one's means of confirming that identity, one's capacity for a sense of cohesiveness about who one is, and one's strategies for maintaining and restoring self-esteem became the dominant categories of analysis, replacing concepts such as drive and defense. The self psychologists and the intersubjective analysts have reframed our understanding of what is central in human psychology to such a degree that early Freudian theory seems a distant relative. For a recent, solidly researched and philosophically rich argument about the development of the self, and about the clinical implications of understanding that process, see Irene Fast's (1998) study of "selving."

As this transformation was affecting mainstream psychoanalysis, paper after paper was written rethinking symptoms and syndromes in terms not of how they managed anxiety but of how they supported critical feelings of self-continuity and self-worth. A prime example is Stolorow's 1975 article on the narcissistic functions of masochism and sadism, phenomena previously understood only in terms of drive and anxiety. In parallel with these developments, psychoanalytic technique was being revised and redefined. Intersubjective theorists and self psychologists emphasized not the therapist's objectivity and interpretation but subjectivity and empathic attunement (Stolorow et al., 1987; Wolf, 1988; Rowe & MacIsaac, 1989; Shane, Shane, & Gales, 1997). Along with these developments in technique came an appreciation of the inevitability of narcissistic injury to the patient during therapy, followed by ideas about how to address such clinical crises of self-esteem when they occurred.

Most practitioners were way ahead of theorists in this area. One learns fast enough as a full-time therapist that if one is not sensitive to the narcissistic requirements of one's patients, one will either lose them or spend most of one's treatment time mopping up after one's empathic failures. In fact, I suspect that Kohut's immediate popularity among therapists in the early 1970s, despite his impenetrable language in *The Analysis of the Self* (1971), derived largely from the fact that he gave an elegant psychoanalytic rationale for doing things that therapists with normal compassion and intuition were already doing, often in defiance of the rather constricting technical training they had been given (though worrying, in many cases, that they were "breaking a rule"—my colleague Stanley Moldawsky refers to this as deference to the "Orthodox Committee" that analysts carry around in their heads). Activities on the therapist's part such as occasional self-disclosure, acceptance of small gifts, and offering support and praise became, in Kohut's formulation, not "parameters" (Eissler, 1953) or "deviations" from technique but important expressions of the practitioner's respect and understanding. "First, preserve the client's self-esteem" is perhaps the best transposition of the Hippocratic principle "First, do no harm" into the psychotherapeutic arena.

CLINICAL IMPLICATIONS OF ASSESSING SELF-ESTEEM

Psychotherapy must concern itself with self-esteem issues in a number of ways. First of all, we must consider whether the person's value system is close enough to our own, or at least comprehensible enough to us, that the two parties to the treatment can work together effectively. Second, as therapists, we must preserve the patient's sense of self-worth enough to keep the treatment going; we must learn how to communicate our ideas in ways that keep injuries to the person's pride to a minimum. Third, we must address the difficult question of how to help patients change the ways they evaluate themselves when the bases of their self-esteem are clearly unrealistic and maladaptive. Fourth, when clients have been reared without an internal gyroscope orienting them toward acts that make them legitimately proud of themselves, we often have to help them define and articulate their values. Fifth, we must figure out how to work with those who bolster their self-esteem in ways that damage others. I now take up these questions.

Do the Requisites of This Person's Self-Esteem Permit Me to Work Effectively with Him or Her?

In our training as therapists, most of us get the implicit message that we should be able to work therapeutically with anyone, or at least with anyone whose type of problem we have been trained to address. Yet a few years of practice is enough for most of us to learn which kinds of people we are good at helping and which kinds we should refer. Some of my colleagues, for example, love working with trauma victims, while others screen them out of their practices. Some are energized by the intensity of clients in the borderline range, while others cannot tolerate the storms of affect these patients unleash. Among my therapist friends are some with a special talent and affinity for schizophrenic people, for the emotionally retarded, for the learning disabled, for geriatric populations. Other colleagues cannot imagine working with people in these categories. These predilections are not just reflective of divergent training experiences and technical competencies. They express core features of therapists' personalities, most notably the different ways they meet their respective individual needs to maintain and restore self-esteem.

One social worker I treated several years ago was remarkably gifted in helping the severely and profoundly retarded, a group of clients not well known for their attractiveness to therapists. We figured out together that the sense of calling she had for this work derived from the damage her self-esteem had suffered when she could not "get through" to her severely depressed, alcoholic mother. By working with a group that virtually everybody regarded as "unreachable," she was repairing her childhood sense of inadequacy and healing her wounded pride. A woman I studied in my research on altruism had made it a vocation to work with the criminally insane, a population not only unappealing to most of us but also dangerous. Her self-esteem structure reflected an identification with her father, a devout Methodist minister, who had repeatedly emphasized Jesus's injunction, "Inasmuch as ye have done it unto one of the least of these my brethren, ye have done it unto me" (Matthew 25: 40). She got great satisfaction from her work, and the inmates loved her.

If we acknowledge that the emotional engine that drives the psychotherapy process in the clinician is the opportunity to support and restore his or her own self-esteem, we can appreciate how problematic it can be for a practitioner to work with someone whose narcissism is based on radically different assumptions from those of the therapist. For example, many psychotherapists cannot work comfortably or effectively with psychopathic patients. The self-esteem of therapists typically depends on their behaving lovingly; therapists tend to reject raw power and financial gain in favor of opportunities to be authentic and connected with others. They may feel deeply disturbed by those who disdain genuineness and attachment and instead require power and wealth to feel positive about themselves. One cannot work well with someone toward whom one feels emotional alienation or contempt, and clinicians who cannot find a power-related area in their own self-esteem economy are better off not working with the antisocial among us. Similarly, many practitioners shun patients with self disorders because the need of a narcissistic person to impress others at all costs grates on the therapist's more internal criteria for self-evaluation or activates the therapist's unconscious shame about his or her own unacknowledged narcissism.

The question of whether one should take on a patient with values and convictions that are significantly different from one's own extends beyond the category of his or her psychopathology. A practitioner who takes pride in his contempt for religious sentimentality should not try to treat someone whose self-esteem depends on maintaining the sense of an intimate connection with God. A therapist for whom sexual fidelity is a primary value will find it hard to understand and enjoy a client whose self-esteem depends on recurrent sexual conquest. A clinician whose narcissism depends on the commitment to offer low fees to clients in need will be a poor match with a patient whose narcissism is dependent on making big money.

These considerations are pertinent not just because the treater's empathy cannot be accessed when he or she and the patient are too different. The client's capacity to identify and make therapeutic use of a clinician is also compromised when there are significant disparities in the self-esteem requirements of the respective parties to the treatment— whether or not the therapist feels any difficulty accepting the patient's values. Let me use myself as an example of this problem. My standard fee has consistently been moderate, and I have also always taken a certain number of patients at low cost. This practice is possible for me because I have a home office, low overhead, and a well-paid spouse. It also reflects the fact that my family of origin was financially comfortable and did not rear me with anxiety about money. But most centrally, it expresses my preference not to limit my practice to the treatment of upper-middle-class and wealthier clients. It is part of my ego ideal, probably related to my coming of age in the affluent and idealistic 1960s, not to be overly greedy, not to chase money above other goods, and not to isolate myself from the opportunity to help people in marginal and disadvantaged groups (certain of my more cynical friends and colleagues have diagnosed masochism here as well; if they are right, it is hopelessly ego-syntonic).

It is not hard for me, however, to appreciate how central money can be to the self-esteem of someone whose historical and current circumstances differ from mine. And for all my efforts to act with generosity, I love having money. It is not a stretch for me to empathize with those who like to accumulate it. So I did not expect to have trouble working with people whose core motivations were more financial than mine. But I found that they had trouble working with me! They assumed that my modest fees meant that I must not be very competent, or that I must *feel* I am not worth much, or that I am incomprehensibly self-defeating, or that I feel morally superior to those who pursue filthy lucre. Eventually, I decided that I should either charge a hefty fee to those for whom personal value and monetary value were closely tied (this was not exactly an agonizing decision), or refer such patients to therapists whose fee and car and office advertise their prosperity.

In other words, I had to come to terms with the fact that it was difficult for some patients to see my fiscal arrangements as representing a simple, nonproblematic difference between us. While this initially surprised me, especially because I assumed they would be happy to save some expense, on reflection, their attitude makes sense to me. Because there was a significant disparity in what supported our respective self-images, financially oriented clients were inevitably in the position of having either to devalue me to maintain their own pride, or, alternatively, to idealize my imputed indifference to money, with the side effect that they would feel morally inferior. This is not a good emotional position from which to begin the collaborative work of therapy.

Research on fees set by private practitioners (Lasky, 1984; Liss-Levinson, 1990) has revealed that my custom and the rationale for it are fairly typical of people of my gender. There is an interesting discrepancy in self-established fees between male and female therapists, one that has been lamented by some as indicating that the self-esteem of most female practitioners is weaker than that of their male colleagues— in other words, if women felt better about themselves, they would charge as much as men. I prefer to understand this sex difference in terms of female emotional realities and derivative self-esteem structure. Women frequently are not paid for work that is universally acknowledged to be valuable. Even ambitious, gainfully employed women who cut back or take time off to rear their children must judge themselves by nonmercenary standards or else feel chronically depressed. I believe the data about gender and fee setting suggest not that most female therapists are self-devaluing, but that their self-esteem is less related to their income than is that of many men (cf. Liss-Levinson, 1990).

The emotional stresses on therapists make it hard to do psychotherapy well. Under ideal circumstances, we have sufficient professional autonomy to make decisions about the nature of our practices. When ideal circumstances do not prevail, the best we can do is depend on self-knowledge to improve our work. One of the reasons for the time-honored rule in psychoanalytic institutes that candidates be analyzed is that the process allows one to get in touch with aspects of one's own personality and self-esteem structure that are not overt. In analysis, ethical, law-abiding people learn to access the part of themselves that admires the criminal; generous people find their greed; sexually conservative people find their lust; those who cherish honesty come face to face with the small deceits they perpetrate on themselves and others. It is not a great leap to understand how someone else could attach significant self-esteem to attitudes that play only a cameo role on one's own personal stage. Even without intensive therapy, one can try to expand access to disowned parts of the self, with the reward that the range of patients one can help increases with every hard-won insight.

How Can I Give Patients Useful Information without Injuring Their Self-Esteem?

Because much of what a therapist says is inherently wounding, he or she must find ways to intervene that preserve a client's self-esteem. All of us suffer at least a wince when someone tells us something about ourselves that we did not already know. We want to learn, but it feels humiliating to be taught. Every psychotherapeutic interpretation is thus a narcissistic injury. The central focus of training in the art of therapy should be how to convey what the client needs to know in order to change, with a minimum of injury to his or her self-esteem. This skill is often called tact (Greenson, 1967), but ordinary tact will not be enough to protect the feelings of some patients, who require a much more specific understanding of what supports their pride and what undermines it.

Classical analytic technique dictates that wherever possible, it should be the client who comes up with insights, who derives interpretations from his or her free associations, dreams, and transference reactions (Strachey, 1934; Fenichel, 1945). The analyst's activity should be limited to clearing away the resistances that keep warded-off knowledge about the self out of consciousness. One reason for this rule is that by observing it, the analyst is less likely to impose a meaning on the patient's material that comes from the analyst's preconceptions rather than the patient's experience. In a well-conducted analysis, both parties should sometimes be surprised by what emerges from the analysand's unconscious (Reik, 1948). But a less-discussed reason for the classical technical position concerns the client's self-esteem. The narcissistic enhancement that occurs when one comes up with one's own understanding compensates for the narcissistic injury of acknowledging that one had not known this already, on one's own.

By elevating attunement and empathy to superordinate roles (e.g., Wolf, 1988; Shane et al., 1997), self psychologically oriented practitioners go even further than the classical analysts in protecting a patient's self-esteem. It is probably not accidental that the self psychology movement picked up steam at a time when practitioners were discovering that more and more clients could not tolerate conventional resistance analysis and the invitation to uncover disowned strivings. All therapists know the shock of making a comment that one expects to be experienced as empathic and supportive and having the client react as if he or she has been sadistically criticized. This phenomenon is particularly noteworthy in patients with narcissistic and borderline psychologies; in fact, such a response has come to be widely understood as a diagnostic flag for those conditions.

The numbers of people with such problems seemed to be swelling—or at least they were coming to therapists with far more frequency—in the second half of the twentieth century (as I have already commented, many aspects of contemporary culture make this phenomenon quite understandable). Unlike neurotic-level clients, whose pain at being told something they have not figured out for themselves is mitigated by their appreciation of the therapist's wish to help, borderline and narcissistic patients simply feel attacked. Accordingly, a lot of our more recent technical literature concerns itself with suggestions about how to reduce this sense of being savagely criticized, how to preserve a client's self-esteem, and how to make reparation when that self-esteem is inevitably injured in the course of the therapist's efforts to understand and help.

The famous shift from a one-person to a two-person psychoanalytic metapsychology in the late twentieth century (Aron, 1990; Mitchell & Black, 1995) was partly motivated by clinical attention to self-esteem issues. When the analyst, instead of adopting the role of the objective outsider on whom the patient's "stuff" is projected, acknowledges participation in and contribution to what goes on between therapist and client, the client carries less of the burden of shame over what happens between them. One reason the intersubjectivists stress so much the co-construction of the transference and the two-person nature of every interaction is that the potential for injury to a patient's self-esteem is considerably reduced when the analyst takes responsibility for his or her contribution to the difficult emotional states that arise in therapy.

In addition to the technical suggestions of those in the self psychology and intersubjective camps, there are numerous helpful resources for therapists who want to learn how to share potentially useful information with patients without damaging their self-esteem. Recent writing on supportive therapy (e.g., Pinsker, 1997), on therapy with borderline and narcissistic clients (e.g., Meissner, 1984; Kernberg, Selzer, Koenigsberg, Carr, & Appelbaum, 1989), and on the treatment of people with substance-abuse problems (Levin, 1987; Richards, 1993) is rich with ideas on how the therapist can promote change while minimizing wounds to the patient. Lawrence Josephs's (1995) *Balancing Empathy and Interpretation* contains a particularly useful discussion of the technical challenges one faces when one tries to help someone with both character pathology and fragile self-esteem. Finally, Sue Elkind (1992) has written a valuable book on the process of consulting to therapeutic dyads when they cannot get beyond the stalemates that hurt feelings create.

In addition to referring the reader to texts such as these, let me offer one illustration of a technical procedure that emanates from the assessment that one's client has significant problems with self-esteem. One way to communicate potentially hurtful but ultimately important ideas to a person with marked narcissistic vulnerability is to package an intervention in such a way that the patient feels not just criticized but also admiringly accepted. Such comments must be genuine if they are not to be taken as hollow and manipulative, but usually it is easy for a therapist to find things about the client that are realistically praiseworthy. For example, I often find myself saying things like, "You're such an interesting person. On the one hand, you're so accomplished and articulate, and on the other, you can get completely paralyzed in certain situations." Or, "I would never know if I met you socially how much anxiety you carry around. Your outward demeanor is very self-assured, and the only way I know how much fear you suffer is that you tell me about it." Such statements are intended to counteract shame, to avoid the injury that would occur if I simply observed, even with sympathy and tact, "You get very paralyzed sometimes," or "Anxiety is a big problem for you."

It is useful in such interventions to know on what specific foundations the patient's self-esteem is built. A woman who prides herself on being smart can accept attention to her shortcomings if her intellect is simultaneously recognized ("For a person of such high intelligence, it must be frustrating that you can't resolve these emotional difficulties with brainpower alone"). A man who needs to see himself as possessed of a subtle, exquisite sensibility can often own up to his own contribution to his unhappiness if his sensitivity is explicitly acknowledged in the process ("It might not bother a less sensitive person to have these marital problems, but for you it's important to face them"). The assessment of what supports the self-esteem of an individual person thus has very concrete, practical implications for technique.

How Can I Modify This Person's Maladaptive Self-Esteem Pattern?

Very often, the reason someone has come for treatment involves his or her inability to abandon an established reservoir of self-esteem despite life circumstances that no longer feed it. We are all familiar with the former football hero who has not made the transition to other ways of feeling important, and who substitutes boozy reminiscences of his glory days for activities that would make him feel good about himself on some grounds other than his athletic prowess. Another cultural stereotype with some basis in reality is that of the former beauty who, as she ages, sinks into depression or drugs because her self-esteem has been entirely dependent on her youthful attractiveness. Sometimes, as therapists, we are aware of working preventively to expand a young person's sources of self-esteem so that as he or she moves along in life, the lost role of ingenue or brilliant-young-guy-on-the-way-up or athletic whiz or sexpot will be replaced by more durable sources of pride.

Sometimes just the accidents of life destroy a person's otherwise effective strategies for feeling positive self-regard. One woman I worked with had a history that contributed to her pinning her self-esteem on extreme helpfulness and conscientiousness. Her mother, who was one of several children in a family of limited resources, had been designated on the basis of her intelligence as one of the kids who would go to college. Then she became pregnant with my patient. The family solution was that my client should be reared by her mother's sister, who, seen as less brainy, then married sooner than she otherwise would have in order to provide an intact family for the baby. As a child, this woman felt keenly that her existence had created a terrible problem for her birth mother and then had burdened her aunt. In addition, the truth about her birth was kept from the children her aunt and uncle (whom she referred to as her mother and father) subsequently had, leaving her to feel alone with a shameful secret. It became pivotal to her self-esteem that she take care of others, ask for nothing for herself, and prove that her presence on the planet could be an asset rather than a drain.

This solution to her childhood dilemma worked fairly well for her until her mid-fifties. She was a devoted mother, a reliable neighbor, a conscientious friend, and most pertinent to this vignette, an exemplary employee of the large corporation for which she worked. She had felt reasonably good about herself for most of her adult life. When she came to me, however, she was practically at death's door from the stress of trying to deal with a new boss. She was exhausted, despairing, and suffering panic attacks with heart pain and palpitations that two physicians thought might indicate or lead to heart pathology as well. After almost thirty years of valued service, she had been caught in a downsizing operation in which a hatchet woman had been brought in to get rid of the most costly employees (this was not her paranoid interpretation of her circumstances; I had information from other sources that this was in fact the case). Her new superior kept finding fault with everything she did, and the harder she worked, the more nitpicking was the criticism. Her old ways of proving her value just did not work in a system that wanted her out, and she could not shift the basis of her self-esteem to some other means of coping—such as scaling down her production and trying to hide out, or organizing with other employees, or bringing a lawsuit, or simply leaving for a better job. She just kept working harder. A major challenge to the therapy was helping her find self-esteem in areas other than sacrificing herself to the insincere and insatiable demands of her supervisor.

This client had a somewhat self-sacrificing personality structure that was no problem to her as long as the authorities in her life were more or less benign. As is frequently the case when people seek therapy, fate had thrown her a situation that her habitual defenses gave her no help in handling. In addition to appreciating the defenses involved, one way of understanding a self-defeating character structure is in terms of its self-esteem requirements: People who are characterologically masochistic attach their pride to self-sacrifice and care for others. Most personality disorders can be similarly described by the way people in a given category pursue self-esteem. For example, the psychopathic person becomes pumped up by excitement and power; the narcissistic person basks in validation and admiration from others; the schizoid person aspires to creative authenticity; the depressive person covets basic acceptance by, and closeness to, others; the obsessive–compulsive person seeks a sense of control.

It is dangerous, especially in a rapidly changing world, for individuals to hang their self-regard on only one hook. In working with people who have inflexible personalities, clinicians try, either intuitively or self-consciously, to expand the criteria by which their clients derive self-esteem. Thus, we attempt to make the antisocial person capable of pride in honesty, the narcissistic person responsive to an internal voice, the schizoid person pleased with a tolerance for ordinary social hypocrisies, the depressive person proud of risking anger, the masochistic person capable of relishing self-assertion; the obsessive–compulsive person gratified with a growing ability to go with the flow. We endeavor to make people aware of attitudes they can access that are dystonic to their main ways of valuing themselves. Even beyond that, we try to help them enjoy and take pride in these inclinations (Silverman, 1984; Hammer, 1990).

This is not easy. When a person's core principles are challenged, he or she is just as likely to think that the therapist is morally corrupt as to consider becoming more flexible. Questioning a person's internalized standards amounts to criticizing the early love objects whose ideas that person assimilated, internalized caregivers from whom increased psychological separation feels alien and even dangerous. In order to suggest ways of expanding access to self-esteem, a therapist usually has to communicate first just how deeply he or she appreciates the client's efforts to feel pride and avoid shame by time-tested methods. "It seems very important to you to feel in control," or "You seem to feel quite devastated when you are not appreciated," are the kinds of comments by which a therapist communicates understanding of a patient's self-esteem system. Even in these simple reflections, though, there is an implicit message: "It is possible not to need so much control and still feel okay," and "It is possible to bounce back faster from the disappointment of being unacknowledged." In the language of Freud's structural theory, the patient is being encouraged to make alien to his or her superego something that has been syntonic to it. The process by which clients develop some objectivity about their personal economies of self-esteem is slow, but one of the most positive outcomes of good treatment is a more resilient self-esteem, one that can draw from many sources.

A common clinical experience is working with a depressive person who has made it a condition of his or her self-esteem to think only "nice" thoughts and have only "nice" feelings. "Isn't that terrible?" such a client will ask, after confessing to some very ordinary thought-crime, such as the wish that her mother-in-law would drop dead. In these instances, therapists have to do a fairly aggressive kind of education: Feelings and thoughts hurt no one; it is normal to have hostile attitudes; the only reasonable basis for judging oneself involves how one acts, not how one feels subjectively; if we were all judged by our private and transient wishes, there would be a serious overpopulation problem in Hell.

In addition, it helps for the therapist to challenge the superego in a teasing way: "Oh. I forgot. You're too *nice* to have hostile feelings toward someone who's been nasty to you." This sometimes evokes anger—not a bad thing. The therapist's welcoming of an angry response gives the patient an opportunity to learn that the expression of a negative feeling can produce increased intimacy, that genuineness feels better than niceness and does not necessarily provoke rejection. The client may feel attacked, but note that what is under assault is not the total person but his or her self-attacking tendency. This kind of support seems much more effective with depressive people than positive feedback and education alone. When someone has a perverse standard for feeling self-esteem, the therapist's slightly sarcastic questioning of that standard, provided it occurs once there is a good working relationship, can be rather dramatically therapeutic.

How Can I Help This Patient Create a Reasonable Basis for Self-Esteem?

Analysts have noted for decades that it is easier to soften an overzealous superego than to strengthen a weak one. Patients whose self-esteem derives from unrealistically demanding internal moral standards can be induced over time to be less hard on themselves. They identify with the therapist's nonjudgmental interest in them. They may soften up via realizing the infantile, all-or-nothing nature of their severe judgments. They may rearrange their self-esteem structure by mellowing out in one area while becoming compensatorily more demanding elsewhere—for example, in analytic therapy, many patients counteract the narcissistic injury inherent in owning their "selfishness" with a sense of pride in becoming more honest with themselves. On the other hand, when someone's self-esteem derives from transient pleasures and excitements that have no staying power, or from foiling authorities, or from heaping blame on others, it is hard for a therapist to help the patient transfer the pursuit of self-esteem into areas where there is some chance for long-term self-regard. A difficult aspect of working with narcissistically oriented and impulsive people is that their ways of feeling good about themselves are ultimately unsatisfying and self-defeating, and yet they cannot imagine other ways of pursuing enjoyment.

"If it feels good, do it" is not a very effective long-term recipe for a gratifying life. Many people in our culture, presumably engaged in the pursuit of happiness that the Declaration of Independence endorses, believe that if they only get enough of what they want, they will feel good about themselves. In fact, it is one of the important findings of psychoanalytic investigation that our desires are both boundless and conflictual. It follows that the way to feel satisfaction with one's life is not via accumulation (of goods or experiences or fame), since we will never have "enough," but to find ways to enjoy what we have. Not to put too puritanical a slant on things, the capacity for delay of gratification has its rewards. Renouncing something we think would compromise us morally creates more long-term self-esteem than going for the quick thrill.

The effort to get one's self-esteem from external sources, in the absence of internal ones, constitutes an orientation to life that dooms the patient to a series of empty adventures with no potential for lasting emotional gratification and pride. Patients themselves know this at some level. Narcissistically organized people tend to seek therapy in their forties or later, when they begin to feel the hollowness of the way they have structured their lives. Even antisocial people have been known to mature into more or less law-abiding citizens if they survive their reckless youth. The emphasis put by twelve-step programs on a connection with God suggests widespread appreciation of the fact that one cannot change from a psychology of impulsivity to one of self-control without internalizing an image of moral authority.

The hypersensitivity of narcissistically organized people to criticism makes it very hard for therapists to suggest means other than the ones they already use by which they can avoid shame and feel pride. Still, it can plant a seed for a therapist to say, on being told by a patient that he has walked out on a job without notice because he did not feel like working anymore, "That must feel good. But what about your self-esteem? Wouldn't you feel better about yourself if you had stuck it out for a while?" Notice that the therapist is putting the issue of self-evaluation under the patient's control rather than offering his or her direct criticism of the person's behavior.

How Can I Reorient This Person's Self-Esteem to Reduce Destructiveness to Others?

Some people with more severe narcissistic pathology, most psychopathic people, and most addicts (of various kinds) not only harm their own prospects for the good life but also do damage to others. It is part of the therapist's job with such patients to help them find sources of self-esteem in socially positive areas. Cognitive-behavioral therapists try to do this, for example, with procedures such as anger management training and empathy training. From a psychoanalytic standpoint, the point to such therapies is not only to get problematic behaviors under control but also to create an atmosphere in which patients want to identify with values and standards for self-esteem that have not previously been effectively transmitted; that is, therapy should produce a modification of internal structures regulating self-esteem.

The success of twelve-step programs where traditional therapies fail may be partly due to their supplying a set of explicit values and bases for self-esteem support to people whose histories were deficient in them. In traditional therapies, the clinician tries not to inflict his or her values on the patient—a position that is fine for those patients who have reliable values but that amounts to professional neglect with those who lack them. The appeal to many people of cults and strict religious denominations also attests to a longing among many rudderless individuals for a clear, authoritative statement of what is good and bad, what should make one feel positive about oneself, and what constitutes a sin or a breach of faith with the community.

For therapists working one-on-one with a voluntary patient whose actions are often destructive to others, it is a tricky business to try to reorient someone toward the socially positive. For a psychopathic person, it is a considerable success to transform a pure power dynamic into a more benign narcissistic one; for example, the person shifts from basing his or her self-esteem on feeling powerful at any cost to basing it on looking good to the community. One man I worked with, who came for therapy after a long career as a drug dealer, was able to change a lifelong destructive pattern by joining a religious community, where he confessed to his previous life of crime and earned the admiration of the flock for his redemption. He found this new status in a nonunderworld culture so gratifying—not to mention so much less likely to send him to jail than his previous style of life—that he was able to keep his behavior reasonably prosocial.

Interpretively, a therapist must move even more slowly with immediate-gratification-oriented clients than with those whose self-esteem requires heroic self-denial. Efforts to build internal sources of self-regard tend to be dismissed by substance-abusing, impulse-ridden or antisocial clients, not entirely without justification, as moralistic and judgmental. When the therapist's interventions are *not* dismissed, patients can feel a shame so great that they bolt from treatment rather than endure another mortification. While conveying a rigorous honesty, the therapist must not sentimentalize good behavior and must find empathy with the morally compromised person's cynicism about what makes the world go round. The focus has to stay on concrete matters such as whether the person is in control, whether he or she has risked looking weak or foolish, whether the behavior under discussion will come back to haunt the client. And, of course, the therapist's own attitude of pride in being ethical, especially if it coexists with a realistic unflappability about the client's contrasting shenanigans, will eventually sink in.

SUMMARY

In this chapter, I have emphasized individual differences in self-esteem: how it is maintained and repaired, how reliable it is, and how reasonable and socially valuable are the standards that support it. I have reviewed psychoanalytic thinking about self-esteem issues, from classical reflections on superego formation through more contemporary emphases on the fate of self-esteem in the bipersonal field of therapy. I have emphasized the significance of understanding a patient's particular narcissistic economy and have explored several clinical issues that depend on such an understanding. These included the match of a given patient with a given therapist, the problem of communicating therapeutically with minimal injury to a person's self-esteem, the modification of maladaptive ways of deriving self-esteem, the treatment of clients who lack the internal basis for experiencing lasting satisfaction with themselves, and the reduction of the destructiveness of those whose self-esteem is purchased at the expense of other people's suffering.

CHAPTER TEN

⟨⟨⟨

Assessing Pathogenic Beliefs

D ESPITE the popular conception that the main concerns of psycho-analysis are drives and emotions, analytic theory has always paid care-ful attention to the cognitive dimension of experience, especially at the unconscious level. If how we think were not central to a psychoanalytic understanding of individual character and pathology, then analytic technique would never have included so much stress on interpretation, on bringing unconscious ideas into consciousness. Freud's original model (e.g., 1911) posited that along with primitive drives and affects, there exists in the unconscious part of the mind a type of mentation that he called "primary process thought," the residue of our earliest, preverbal ways of apprehending our world. This archaic cognitive mode was construed by him as prerational, prelogical, egocentric and wish-driven, that is, governed by the pleasure principle rather than the reality principle. In an interesting anticipation of some of Piaget's work,* Freud stressed the symbolic, visual character of primary process thought, and he emphasized its magical, wish-fulfilling nature. Among the ways he disturbed the Victorian sensibilities of his time were not only his claim that children have sexuality but also his conclusion that regardless of how "civilized" and highly educated we are, remnants of

---

*Freud's theories may have had some direct effects on Piaget's model of cognitive development, a model that played a critical role in dismantling the narrowly behaviorist hegemony in academic psychology and laying the groundwork for the cognitive-behavioral sensibility that now dominates there. Piaget was analyzed by Sabina Spielrein, a hospitalized patient and presumed lover of Carl Jung (Carotenuto, 1983; Kerr, 1993), who became a student and colleague of Freud, and who may have been the source of his original theorizing about a death instinct. This brilliant and creative woman was murdered by the Nazis in 1941. We know about her complex role in the early psychoanalytic movement mainly because of some diaries and letters that survived her.

primitive, self-referential ways of thinking continue to exist in our unconscious life and to control our behavior to a far greater degree than we like to think.

In addition to positing some universal cognitive processes, Freud talked about individual differences in inner convictions and their relationship to people's idiosyncratic psychologies. For example, in his essay "Some Character-Types Met with in Psycho-Analytic Work" (1916), he emphasized the determinative nature of unconscious beliefs. Describing someone who considered himself an "exception" to the rules that should govern others, he emphasized this man's assumption that he was subject to a special divine protection. Freud noted that he had "in his infancy been the victim of an accidental infection from his wet-nurse, and had spent his whole later life making claims for compensation, an accident pension, as it were, without having any idea on what he based those claims" (p. 313). Invoking a similar cognitive explanation in depicting a type of person he labeled a "criminal from a sense of guilt," Freud argued that some people commit misdeeds in order to square their sense of themselves with a *preexisting conviction* that they are transgressive and culpable.

THE NATURE AND FUNCTION
OF PATHOGENIC BELIEFS

Among contemporary psychoanalytic writers and researchers, the ones who have put most emphasis on unconscious pathogenic beliefs are Joseph Weiss and Harold Sampson and the San Francisco Psychotherapy Research Group (e.g., Weiss et al., 1986; Weiss, 1993). Originally labeling their orientation as "control–mastery theory," these investigators found through empirical examinations of successful psychotherapies that understanding a client's core convictions, and then understanding his or her therapeutic engagement as expressing the effort to disprove these convictions, gave a powerful account of the change process in treatment. Sampson and Weiss and their colleagues stress that we all have organizing beliefs, often existing at an unconscious level, that tend to operate like self-fulfilling prophecies. If one has been lucky enough to have internalized beliefs that are benign and adaptive, one has a good chance to live a satisfying life. But if one has internalized beliefs that stress, for example, the badness of the self, or the futility of effort, or the danger of closeness, or the inevitability of betrayal, one is destined to suffer repetitively unless one gets good therapy.

Contemporary psychoanalytic models that stress cognition suggest the exciting possibility of a rapprochement between analytic and cognitive-behavioral sensibilities. The scholarship of Wilma Bucci (1997), to mention only one researcher of distinction in this area, has recently given us reason to hope for an empirically sound integration of cognitive science and psychoanalytic thinking on the theoretical level. As noted earlier, Allen Schore's work (e.g., 1994) suggests that it can be done at the neurobiological level. At the clinical level, there has been for some time a lively interest in psychotherapy integration (e.g., Wachtel, 1977; Arkowitz & Messer, 1984). Lately, interest in a theoretical and technical synthesis has reflected the fact that a mutual interest in cognition unites psychoanalytic and cognitive-behavioral therapists. It has not often been noted that Albert Ellis, Aaron Beck, and other pioneering cognitive therapists are similar to Freud in emphasizing the role of individual irrational beliefs in creating and maintaining psychopathology. According to them, the therapist's main job is to challenge such ideas. Where they have differed from Freud and other psychoanalysts is in their opinion that there is no need to posit a dynamic, unconscious part of the mind where these destructive beliefs reside; they regard them as evocable and addressable without requiring a therapist to assume that mental structure.

Encouragingly to me, some eminent contemporary cognitive-behaviorists (e.g., Barlow, 1998) have noted that recent achievements in brain imaging establish the existence of unconscious processes that must be taken into account in understanding cognition. A few sobering thoughts, however, on the likelihood that individual clinicians will become sophisticated integrators of both psychoanalytic and cognitive-behavioral approaches: Unfortunately, becoming a skilled psychotherapist with an extensive scholarly foundation in either tradition is a long, demanding process, and very few people master a substantial body of literature in both orientations. Matters of personal temperament, the accidents of one's training, and the effectiveness or ineffectiveness of one's personal therapy in either tradition tend to attract a therapist to one or the other approach. Cognitive-behavioral and psychoanalytic positions also contain, respectively, certain irreducible differences of emphasis and assumption (see Messer & Winokur, 1980; Arkowitz & Messer, 1984). Still, it would greatly enrich our field if practitioners of contrasting orientations could appreciate some of the common ground on which psychotherapeutic intervention is based.

Family systems approaches to understanding psychopathology also assume the operation of unconscious beliefs. Family therapists discern these both in individual people and in the phenomenon of the family myth. Ideas such as "If I individuate, Mother will die," or "I have to be the sick one in order to keep my parents from fighting" may characterize the innermost beliefs of the identified patient in a system, while more general ideas such as "If anyone differentiates from the family, we all will be destroyed" may be keeping the identified patient imprisoned in a scapegoat role and the whole family organism stuck in a maladaptive pattern. Systems-oriented practitioners of varying persuasions have developed technologies of intervention designed to disconfirm such beliefs and thereby improve a family's flexibility and growth. Like most cognitive-behavioral clinicians, they tend to be less interested than analytic therapists in whether there is an individual dynamic unconscious, or even whether problematic ideas are admissible to consciousness. If they can be changed via novel experiences, they point out, the family will make progress in treatment.

It is certainly true that the central pathogenic convictions in large numbers of people are not so much unconscious as ego-syntonic. Many clients will readily tell a therapist their organizing assumptions (e.g., "People can't be trusted," "All men are beasts," "Everything I touch turns to shit," "Nobody really gives a damn about other people"). They simply believe these things, and when a treater raises a question about their assumptions, they rush to justify them and to persuade the therapist of their reasonableness. All clinicians have had the experience of thinking they were about to confront a client with something he or she did not know (e.g., "It's as if you believe you don't deserve to take up space on the planet," or "It sounds like you're angry at all authorities, whatever their position") and having the patient reply, "Of course!"— as if the therapist were an idiot for taking so long to see the obvious.

What remains unconscious is sometimes not the belief itself but the interpersonal scenario that created such ideas in the first place. It has been my observation that clients usually cannot change irrational beliefs until they understand where they come from and how they have been operating to protect the self against dangers that no longer exist (more on this later). Freud's young man who saw himself as an exception probably could have told Freud or any other investigator that he felt he was protected by a special providence. What he could not have accessed was his childhood conclusion that this protection was his due because he had already endured his allotted share of suffering, and that it constituted a magical way of avoiding anxieties about his health that were created by his early infection. Presumably, once his adult mind had grasped that this kind of magic made no sense, he could start to renounce his faith in a special personal entitlement.

I want to emphasize here that what we often label "irrational" beliefs are not irrational in the child in whom they originally take form. Young children are inevitably egocentric, in that their knowledge about the world is very limited and depends mainly on their awareness of their own inner state. There is much they do not understand, including the exigencies of having to work for a living, the demands of the larger world outside the home, the impact of political events, the realities of illness and death, the nature of mature sexuality, the vicissitudes of addiction, and, in general, the complex and competing strivings of the adults around them. They do understand their own rather stark and unsubtle feelings, and they generalize from those. They put together the best explanation of their circumstances that they can, given the limits of their information, and they draw the best conclusions available about how to cope with life. Like any conscientious researcher in the logical positivist tradition, they generate the most parsimonious explanation to fit the data.

For example, the little boy whose father disappears when he is three cannot appreciate that his parents got a divorce for reasons unrelated to him, and that his father moved away rather than face his anguish being a visitor in the home where he formerly lived. Instead, the boy concludes that because he was not good enough, his father punished him by leaving. He further concludes that male authorities cannot be trusted, and that he will be safe around them only if he tests their reactions to his badness before he attaches to them. Thus may begin a lifetime of provocation in the hope that some father figure will love him despite his deficiencies. Eventually his pathogenic beliefs may go underground, out of his conscious awareness, but the feelings and behavior associated with them will persist.

Many individuals discover their pathogenic convictions only in the controlled regression of a psychoanalytic treatment, or in the shock of a comparably transformative experience (for instance, in the wake of falling in or out of love, after being moved by a play, or from experiencing another state of consciousness—drug-induced or otherwise achieved). In such circumstances, people are amazed to find that "at some level" they believe numerous illogical things. One of my patients, for example, was astounded to learn that he had been unconsciously blaming his father for the death of his mother from an aneurysm when he was eight years old. A colleague of mine described coming to the upsetting realization that she believed ("in my gut—not my head") that women who compete with men will be destroyed. I remember my own mortification on discovering during my analysis, very much without my analyst's suggestion to that effect, that I had internalized certain ethnic stereotypes that I consciously abhorred.

People's deepest and most irrational convictions about life are famously stubborn. Simply from a learning theory point of view, it is axiomatic that something once thoroughly learned and then intermittently reinforced is deeply resistant to extinction. And intermittent reinforcement is inevitable in a complex world, where all kinds of life experiences will occur. Add to that the phenomenon of the self-fulfilling prophecy (Rosenthal, 1966) or, in psychoanalytic parlance, the operation of projective identification—that is, the fact that people who expect certain kinds of results tend to provoke what they expect—and it is even more understandable how entrenched a pathogenic conviction can be. It is a wonder that in psychotherapy these overdetermined infantile beliefs can be modified at all.

Central to the task of modifying them is the therapist's getting it right about what are the main maladaptive cognitions of any individual person. As with affect, it is easy to project onto someone else the kinds of primitive, self-referential ideas that we have discovered in ourselves rather than to do the disciplined work of discerning that person's idiosyncratic orienting assumptions. For example, a guilt-dominated therapist working with a guilt-ridden client may be doing him or her a great favor in attacking an imputed conviction that everything that goes wrong is one's own fault. In this case, the therapist's psychology is an asset in understanding the patient, who is similar to the clinician. But if the client is not motivated by guilt and instead nurses the problematic attitude that everything that goes wrong is someone else's fault, the therapist who misunderstands that and challenges that person's presumed unconscious self-blame has only reinforced the client's pathological disposition to evade responsibility.

In concluding this section, I want to stress that some pathogenic belief systems are quite complicated and not reducible to a one-line description. Conflict can be a central and confusing feature of them. For example, many schizophrenic people believe that they will be annihilated if they are too separate from other people, but they also believe they will be engulfed if they are too close to them (Karon & VandenBos, 1981). Clients with borderline personality organization are famous for provoking contradictory inferences in those who try to deal with them. Some professionals assume that their central maladaptive belief is "No one will be there for me," while others believe that it is "I can manipulate anyone into being there" (consequently, it is typical in agencies for some staff members to be pleading for indulgence of the borderline patient's wishes and others to be strident about limit setting). Typically, both pathogenic ideas are held by the borderline client, in dynamic conflict, and both sides of the person's inclinations must be dealt with if treatment is to succeed (cf. Masterson, 1976). Therapists who are attentive only to one dimension of the pathogenic ideology of a borderline patient will either reinforce regression or provoke intransigent opposition.

DEVELOPING HYPOTHESES
ABOUT PATHOGENIC BELIEFS

An interviewer trying to understand a person's pathogenic ideas is not usually offered a straightforward account of the client's deepest and most problematic convictions. Even with people whose maladaptive beliefs are ego-syntonic, the therapist may find out about them only by accident. For example, one of my patients had been in treatment for three years before I learned that she confidently believed she had been taking care of me all that time, saving me from the depression that she maintained all female caregivers suffer if they are not lovingly nurtured by the women around them. Only in the most severely paranoid patients are irrational beliefs announced and defended more or less without self-consciousness, and in these cases, such ideas are properly considered delusions. In order to understand the pathogenic cognitions of less damaged clients, one can make inferences based on their general comments about life, on their descriptions of their histories, on their repetitive behavior, and on their transference reactions.

General Comments about Life

The value of simply listening carefully, in an intake interview and later, cannot be overstated. Sometimes in people's parenthetical remarks there is a wealth of information about their inner convictions. For example, a comment such as, "I should have known better than to trust him" implies that the act of trust was going against some inner voice that was counseling distrust. Generalizations such as "Every time I look forward to something, I get disappointed" are likely to be expressing not only an objective reflection on recent events but also a deeper belief that by anticipating something with pleasure, one is magically dooming it to be frustrating. A woman who had been badly neglected as a child once remarked to me, "You talk as if it's the norm for parents to be interested in their kids."

One man I worked with had a very ego-syntonic belief that every time things went well for him, they would then reverse themselves, and he would be punished for having taken pleasure in the good times. His solution to the problem this belief created for him was to attempt not to feel good about anything in the first place. I was clued into this dynamic by his passing remark, "Nothing good comes without a cost." I will say more about him shortly. Another patient of mine used to begin most of his sessions with the comment, "Well, life still sucks." Behind this observation, it turned out, lurked an inner conviction that there was nothing he could do to make life more interesting or gratifying, and that only an omnipotent authority could change things for him. And furthermore, if I, the putative omnipotent authority at hand, was not transforming his life to his satisfaction, it was not because I was relatively impotent to do so, but because I did not care enough about him to exert the effort.

Descriptions of Individual Histories

Very often, even without a relatively dramatic, repetitive behavioral pattern such as these, a client's personal history will suggest the kind of unconscious conclusions that he or she may have drawn from early experience. The interviewer's empathy with the inevitably egocentric explanatory set of the young child helps in trying to infer a particular client's possible pathogenic ideas. Most adopted children, for example, develop at least one theory about why their birth parents rejected them. Girls brought up in families where boys were desired and valued, and boys reared by parents who wanted girls, tend to have strong beliefs to the effect that it is much better to be the other sex (sometimes unconscious, sometimes conscious and rationalized). People who have suffered early and repeated separations from primary objects tend to believe not only that anyone they love will leave them, but also that it is their own badness that will alienate and drive away those they love. Members of maltreated social groups draw deeply troubling conclusions that because of their race or ethnicity or gender or sexual orientation, they are somehow irreparably inferior to members of the contrast group with social power.

It is also important to know simple demographic things such as the socioeconomic status and ethnic composition of the patient's family, since different subcultures promulgate different beliefs about relationship, authority, privacy, gender, intimacy, trust, discipline, and other basic human concerns. Knowledge of a person's religious upbringing also offers information about what kinds of unquestioned beliefs he or she may hold. For example (see Lovinger, 1984), Protestant families tend to induce guilt in children who stay too dependent and fail to act self-reliantly and with the courage of their individual convictions (like Martin Luther, defying the Roman Catholic establishment of his era). Jewish families, in contrast, for whom the maintenance and survival of their community has historically been a critical concern, tend to create guilt in children who go too far afield from the family. Thus, Protestant patients tend to criticize themselves when they feel they have been weak, self-indulgent, and insufficiently independent, while Jewish patients blame themselves for not being caring enough, connected enough, or sensitive enough to others.

In dealing with people who come from ethnic and religious traditions with which the therapist is unfamiliar, the clinician needs to learn about those cultures and their orienting beliefs, both from outside sources and from the patient (Sue & Sue, 1990). I have never known a client who did not appreciate my frank admission of how little I knew about his or her community of origin and feel respected by my wanting to be taught about it. This observation also applies to one's learning in depth from patients about the unique cultures and ideologies of the associations in which they are currently involved. Because people are attracted to groups that embody their preexisting ideas, present-day commitments also contain information about deep-rooted early beliefs. (A fringe benefit of investigating this is the therapist's education. I have been usefully instructed by clients about many areas of life that would have remained relatively invisible to me without their tutelage. These have included the Sufi movement, Quakerism, Buddhism, twelve-step programs, support communities for people with various chronic diseases, and the worlds of animal rights activists, military personnel, motorcycle gangs, acting students, police officers, Christian missionaries, and other groups that promulgate and reinforce particular dogmas.)

The political attitudes of the client and his or her family of origin also afford information about the person's underlying beliefs. For example, American liberals tend to idealize generosity and mercy, while conservatives idealize control and justice (MacEdo, 1991). Some people's personal politics are infused with the conviction that one must resist authority, while others emphasize the social need for compliance and order, and are horrified by rebellious acts. Such attitudes tell a great deal about the underlying lessons the patient has derived from his or her particular history.

Repetitive Behavior

In many people, problematic inner convictions must be discerned from the patient's recurring behavior patterns. For example, one man I worked with was repeatedly, and from my perspective, compulsively, unfaithful to his wife. His explanation for his behavior was that he simply adored women—he was a connoisseur of female beauty and could not resist treating both himself and his attractive admirers to the delights of a sexual affair. The pain he brought to both his spouse and his lovers, when he abandoned each of them in turn for the next exciting conquest, was to his way of thinking a small price they paid for the pleasure of having been connected to a man as appreciative as he was of their charms. It was not hard for me to surmise that he felt a lot of unconscious hostility toward women, though it took him a long time to find and fully experience that aspect of himself. His hostility derived from a personal history in which his mother had abandoned him as a youngster, and because he unconsciously believed that abandonment was inevitable when one becomes attached to a feminine object, he connected and then disconnected himself with subsequent women before it could happen to him again. He was only able to stop misusing women when he understood the relationship between his childhood inference and his behavior.

Another patient of mine had the habit of regarding every choice he had made as the wrong one. He would typically agonize about each important decision (which woman to go out with, which course to take, which job to pursue, which place to go on vacation, and so forth). Once he finally got himself to decide, he became convinced that the road not traveled had been the right road, and he would sink into misery over his bad judgment. We eventually figured out together that underneath this pattern lay at least three pathogenic beliefs: (1) that he would be punished for exerting autonomy, unless he punished himself first; (2) that he did not deserve to enjoy the positive consequences of his choices; and most important, (3) that there is such a thing as a perfect decision, a direction without ambivalence, and the fact that he was not feeling unambivalent about his eventual choice meant that he had been wrong to make it.

This man also had the conviction, as previously noted, that whenever things went well, one should be wary about enjoying them, because they were bound to turn disastrous. I remember intervening rather aggressively with him about the magical thinking underlying this idea, arguing that fortune may rise and fall, but there is no evidence that it falls *because* one has let oneself enjoy its occasional rises. Despite the fact that, as an adult, his pathogenic ideas caused him to suffer greatly—or more accurately, to avoid numerous opportunities for pleasure by turning them into misery—he found himself maddeningly reluctant to give up the sense of being able to exert an omnipotent mind control over the normal exigencies of life.

Transference Reactions

In traditional, long-term treatment, pathogenic ideas reveal themselves slowly in a transference relationship. When they emerge, they often surprise both parties with their intensity. Traumatized people, for example, generally reach a point in therapy when they have an overwhelming conviction that the therapist is about to abuse them. One woman I worked with in analysis—a very high-functioning, realistic person—could not talk to me at a sensitive point in the treatment without curling up into fetal position on the couch as if to protect her vital organs from attack. Her father had been subject to fits of temper in which he lashed out at her physically, striking whatever part of her was within reach.

Depressive people, who carry the inner conviction that their badness will alienate anyone who gets to know them well, typically go through periods of torment in therapy during which they are sure that the clinician is about to reject them. One of my clients in this state of mind found herself begging me not to terminate her treatment, even though she had deliberately chosen me as an analyst on the basis of my reputation for hanging in with patients over the long haul ("I know you tend to stick with people, but they're not me. I keep assuming with each new thing you learn that that will be the last straw, and you'll throw me out in disgust").

When one is not in a position to do analysis or long-term analytic therapy, one must make leaps of inference that are not necessary when pathogenic beliefs can emerge at their own pace. These leaps are important to make intelligently, because the more accurately one apprehends a patient's particular ideology, the more clout one has to influence it. Small transference indications of pathogenic ideas may be apparent at the outset of a therapeutic relationship. The questions a patient asks, the ways in which he or she makes or avoids eye contact, the spirit in which issues like the schedule, the fee, and the cancellation policy are discussed—all suggest the kinds of ideas about relationship that the person brings to the therapy encounter. For example, a comment such as "I only want short-term therapy" may reflect more than a person's concerns about time and expense; they may indicate a pathogenic belief to the effect that if one lets oneself depend, one will be too vulnerable to another person's potentially malevolent power.

CLINICAL IMPLICATIONS OF UNDERSTANDING PATHOGENIC BELIEFS

The importance of making reasonable hypotheses about a person's pathogenic beliefs as early as the first meeting lies in the fact that, from the outset, the patient is unconsciously looking to the therapist to disconfirm the convictions that have compromised and burdened his or her efforts to live a gratifying life (Weiss, 1993). Whether or not it will be part of the work for the practitioner to make interpretations of the client's presumed pathogenic ideas, it is important for the therapist, especially in early sessions, to take pains not to reinforce a person's maladaptive beliefs (in later sessions, once the therapeutic alliance is solid, the inevitable ways in which such cognitions feel temporarily confirmed to the patient can be analyzed and repaired). If a man has been reared by attentive caregivers, he is likely to regard silent attentiveness in the therapist as supportive, but if he has been brought up with negligence and lack of concern, silence will feel to him like indifference. A woman who unconsciously believes that men do not care about her will be relieved to talk to a male therapist who conveys warmth, but a woman brought up by an overinvolved and seductive father may misunderstand that attitude as a threat to her boundaries.

In anxiety disorders and phobic conditions, the pathogenic beliefs that make a situation "irrationally" frightening to a patient are sometimes obvious to a clinician and sometimes more subtle. In order to devise a treatment plan, whether it involves behavioral desensitization or psychodynamic mastery or both, it is essential to know the exact nature of the pathogenic beliefs attached to a feared situation. One agoraphobic woman I worked with felt that what essentially terrified her about going out was the possibility that she would be seen by others as a nervous wreck and would hence become an object of scorn to her acquaintances. As we worked together, it became clear to us that a much more disturbing possibility at the unconscious level was that she might not be noticed at all. Thus, we concluded that she needed to desensitize herself not to negative attention but to lack of attention. (Freud would have noted that fears often conceal wishes: There was an exhibitionistic wish, a wish to be seen and known, behind her fear that others would scrutinize her so critically.) Given the extreme negligence of her alcoholic childhood caregivers, not being noticed had the meaning to her of being exposed to life-threatening dangers. Working with her on a graduated program of being around total strangers who had no interest in her proved to be a better treatment plan than trying to desensitize her to the possible criticism of those who knew her.

There has been a longstanding argument in the psychoanalytic literature about whether it is possible to have a "corrective emotional experience" (Alexander, 1956) that produces lasting change without a full analysis of all the elements of that experience. An ancestor of this argument was a disagreement between Freud and Ferenczi in the early

1900s about whether patients could be essentially reparented, and a relative of it has resurfaced in recent debates between more relationally and more classically oriented analysts discussing the relative therapeutic roles of enactment versus interpretation (see Mitchell & Black, 1995). Whatever their position on this issue, most analytic treaters try assiduously to act in contradiction to the patient's pathogenic expectations, only to find themselves redefined by the patient as confirming those expectations. Such is the power of transference. But no one argues that one should not try to represent a corrective position, whether or not the transference will have to be fully analyzed before it can be assimilated by the client.

We all wish it were easier than it is to change pathogenic ideas. Many people were moved by the portrayal of a psychotherapy relationship in the movie *Good Will Hunting,* when the therapist kept repeating to a young man abused in childhood, "It's not your fault!" The audience response to this scene reveals the extent to which ordinary people appreciate the fact that irrational negative beliefs about the self are, under conditions of childhood mistreatment, both inevitable and intrinsically implicated in a person's psychopathology, and that an attack on them is a fundamental aspect of mental health treatment. Therapists can only wish, however, that our job were as simple as reiterating information that challenges the patient's beliefs. If people were able to reevaluate their pathogenic ideas simply because someone energetically opposed them, there would be no need for psychotherapy. Most of us do not lack for friends, relatives, and authorities who are happy to confront us on our irrationalities, yet we cling to our personal myths as recalcitrantly as a young child clings to a blanket or a teddy bear.

I have already argued that irrational beliefs are more subject to influence if they are conscious. The therapist must not only act differently from the problematic objects in the patient's history, he or she must also help the person to see what expectations are being brought to the relationship. Only then can the patient notice that they are being disconfirmed. Otherwise, people have an uncanny ability to do the information-processing equivalent of putting new wine in old bottles. For example, when a well-meaning therapist tells a depressed woman, "You feel as if there's something terribly bad about yourself, but you're really a very nice person," the patient is much more likely to decide that the therapist is a nice person (in contrast to herself), or that the therapist is a fool to buy into the patient's masquerade as a nice person, than to reconsider her belief that there is something terrible about her essential self. When a therapist lowers the fee for a paranoid man who thinks that the only thing practitioners are interested in is money, the patient is more likely to fear that the therapist is trying to seduce him into a long and expensive dependency than he is to reevaluate his suspicions of others' pecuniary motives.

There are at least three reasons why knowledge of the conditions that gave rise to particular pathogenic beliefs expedite the process of making them conscious and changing them: (1) Patients who know the childhood origins of cherished but ultimately detrimental beliefs can differentiate better between current and prior realities and then evaluate whether the cherished cognitions spawned by the former still have relevance; (2) patients who know why they generated a particular personal ideology feel less crazy in admitting irrational ideas; and (3) patients who appreciate how much infantile dread the maladaptive beliefs have contained will be better able to tolerate the amount of anxiety they will face when they try to act on the basis of contrasting assumptions. When people feel deeply understood in their irrationality and can identify with a therapist's compassion for their having developed their illogical convictions, they can bring much less defensiveness to the task of taking risks that will potentially disconfirm them.

I firmly believe, along with the eloquent Bertram Karon (1998), that these observations apply with no equivocation to the treatment of individuals with delusions. Schizophrenic people who come to understand the childhood origins of their most cherished delusional ideas are in fact able to give them up—once they have enough support to live through the terrors that accompany the effort to change. My own clinical experience attests to this, as does that of many colleagues I know well who have, in defiance of the current enthusiasm for simply medicating and "managing" psychotic patients, devoted themselves to understanding the disturbing subjective world of the severely mentally ill and to giving psychotic clients the empathic interest and devotion that any suffering human being ought to be able to expect from a professional.

I want to talk here briefly about the model that Weiss and Sampson and their colleagues have contributed to our work as therapists. Unlike many clinical theories, it derives not only from practitioner experience but also from empirical investigations of extensive psychoanalyses and therapies, and from interviews with patients and ex-patients. As a result, their inferences are patient-centric rather than analyst-centric. In other words, our prevailing theories about technique (e.g., Greenson, 1967; Etchegoyen, 1991) have described the therapy process from the treater's perspective. They have assumed that the patient wants consciously to change but resists doing so because of deep, unconscious fears about what will happen if change is attempted. Consequently, the therapist must slowly remove such resistance by analyzing it. This is, in fact, how the therapy process feels from the clinician's perspective: I want to help this person to change faster than he or she seems to be able to manage it, so I have to address the part of this person that is opposing my efforts. To the therapist, the forces in the way of change often feel greater than the forces that support it, because those are the dynamics against which the treater battles.

Members of the San Francisco Psychotherapy Research Group have talked about the same dialectic of the wish and fear to change, but from the patient's point of view—a point of view that essentially reverses the emphasis. They see the client as not only wanting to change but also as having a plan by which change can be made. That plan, which has conscious and unconscious elements, includes an effort to disconfirm pathogenic beliefs that the patient knows are problematic but feels as deeply powerful. Thus, the client's point of view is something like: I know that I need my therapist to show me that my deepest convictions are irrational, so I have to keep devising ways to test out whether I can safely abandon them. I want to change faster than I dare, and this process will give me the courage to do it. To the patient, the forces on the side of change are taken for granted, and the inhibitions to change are troubling but not overwhelming.

Passing Tests

According to this way of thinking, doing analytic psychotherapy amounts to passing a succession of the patient's tests. Sampson and Weiss have specified that such tests come in two varieties, the transference test and the passive-into-active transformation (cf. Racker's [1968] concepts of concordant and complementary countertransference, the affective counterparts of these processes). In the first type of test, the client checks out whether the therapist will act like the early object who created the basis for his or her pathogenic beliefs; in the second, the client treats the therapist as he or she felt treated as a child, and then observes closely to see whether the therapist can handle the situation without recourse to the convictions the client developed to cope with that kind of treatment.

Let us consider, for example, the therapeutic situation of a woman who was criticized in deeply hurtful ways by an irritable and autocratic father, and who, as a result, became convinced that the best way to deal with faultfinding authorities is to regard the self as deserving of criticism and to acquiesce. In treatment, such a person might either (1) find herself worrying that the therapist is critical, or (2) criticize the therapist as her father used to criticize her. In either case, she is hoping to see behavior that reflects different underlying ideas from the ones she constructed as a young girl. In the former instance, to be therapeutic, the clinician usually needs only to comment on how the client is experiencing the treater as if he or she were the critical father. The fact that the therapist is quietly inquiring about this rather than acting like a judgmental authority will help the client distinguish between her childhood experience and this new one. In the latter case, the therapist must react nondefensively to the woman's provocation yet without buying into the idea that the client has exposed the practitioner's essential defectiveness. The former is an interpretive intervention; the latter, an enactment.

When Sampson and Weiss were originally marketing control–mastery theory to the larger psychoanalytic community, they were very astute politically. Most of the illustrations they gave of practitioners' therapeutic disconfirmation of patients' pathogenic beliefs involved instances in which disconfirmation was possible without the therapist's deviation from widely accepted technical norms. By this strategy, they avoided alarming conventional practitioners about "wild" or undisciplined interventions. Here is a prosaic example of a treatment situation in which a therapist can pass a patient's test via traditional technique: A man with the pathogenic belief that he is singularly entitled, that others should simply extend themselves to him, is salutarily challenged by the therapist's insistence on regular payment. A more subtle illustration: A woman with the unconscious conviction that she can manipulate information out of anyone, and that she needs to do so for her safety, is well served by the classical position that the therapist discloses as little as possible of a personal nature. Many clients do rethink their irrational convictions in response to a clinician's conservative use of time-honored psychotherapeutic techniques. Aspects of traditional style, such as the therapist's nonjudgmental listening, caring, and remembering, for example, may in themselves diminish pathogenic beliefs about the dangers of being honest.

There are individuals, however, for whom technical options very different from the preceding ones would be the therapeutic choice. A man who is obsessionally preoccupied with paying every debt on time, so that he never feels beholden to anyone, might be deeply helped by a therapist who could tolerate his running up a small bill (and then analyzing his misery and all his catastrophic fantasies about what will happen if he lets someone take care of him this way). A woman who feels she is not entitled to know anything about anybody else might be moved by a therapist who says something like, "You talk a lot about your children and your feelings about being a parent, and yet you've never asked me whether I have kids." The therapist's openness to raising such a question, and his or her willingness to answer it once the patient has explored the meanings of her reluctance to ask any personal questions of the treater, could be a powerful counteractive to the pathogenic belief that she has no right to know anything important about the authorities in her life.

Exposing and Understanding the Beliefs That Produced the Tests

As previously suggested, the clinical implications of understanding a person's pathogenic beliefs are not limited to the therapist's efforts to pass each patient's tests. We also need to help our clients see just what the convictions are that gave rise to the tests, how they originated, how they initially functioned to protect the person, and how they now function to the person's detriment. Otherwise, a lot of clinical progress can be undone once the therapist is no longer around, passing tests. In other words, an examination of the client's underlying maladaptive beliefs is an important part of the working-through process. Even in short-term work, a therapist will accomplish a lot more if he or she not only disconfirms a patient's pathogenic expectations but also comments about the existence and probable childhood significance of those expectations.

An example may illustrate what I mean. Those of us with depressive psychologies respond warmly and with relief to therapists whose behavior invalidates our expectation that we will be rejected if we are fully known. Such expectations are often anchored in childhood experiences of separations in which we concluded that it was *because of our neediness or badness* that we were left. Therapists who limit their antidepressive activity to not rejecting us will feel comforting to us in the short run, but ultimately, they will produce in us not a feeling of self-worth that counteracts our pathogenic beliefs, but an idealization of the therapist for hanging in with such a needy or bad person. And nothing will have happened in such treatments to undermine the magical fantasy supporting such a belief, namely, the hope that if only we can get over our need or become good, we will never have to face abandonment. Unless our self-derogating beliefs and the infantile omnipotent fantasies attached to them are exposed and examined, they will find ways to reassert themselves once the therapy has ended.

Addressing pathogenic ideas is not always a matter for years of psychoanalytic investigation. One man I worked with, whose mother had died of cancer when he was fourteen, was able to do very well after several months of once-per-week therapy in which he discovered in himself the conviction that his mother's death had been the result of his separating emotionally from her. He had come in to work on some boundary problems he felt he had toward his wife, with whom he kept finding himself enmeshed. Once his unconscious guilt had been exposed, he was able to tone it down and realize that his mother would have died whether or not he had accomplished a normal adolescent separation. This discovery allowed him to become more individuated in his marital functioning, more supportive of his wife as a separate person, and less afraid of the possible dire consequences of his "selfishness."

These kinds of insights about the importance of appreciating the lingering effects of the conclusions children draw from their individual predicaments are not limited to the psychoanalytic community. Readers familiar with Jennifer Freyd's (1996) writing on "betrayal trauma" will find very similar arguments, appearing mostly in the language of contemporary cognitive psychology. Freyd stresses how children must, because of their dependent condition, believe that authorities who abuse them are doing so because they deserve it. Otherwise, they would have to face the unbearable terror associated with acknowledging that their survival is in the hands of people who are brutal and untrustworthy. She makes a well-argued, scientifically supported case for understanding memory issues associated with trauma according to formulations such as these, and the relevance of her work to the treatment of traumatized patients is great.

Despite our differing theoretical orientations, I suspect that Freyd and I end up saying rather similar things to victims of childhood physical and sexual abuse:

> "Like all children, you preferred to believe that your abuse derived from something wrong in yourself. Believing this preserved hope for you, in that you could try to figure out what was wrong with you and to change it, and then maybe the abuse would stop. This clinging to hope was preferable to facing the terrifying fact that the people on whom you had to depend were out of control and destructive."

With people who have suffered severe maltreatment in childhood, it is not enough for the therapist to pass transference tests by being nonabusive and to pass passive-into-active tests by refusing to be demoralized by the patient's abuse. In addition to those activities, practitioners must help the client unearth and deconstruct the powerful cognitions that are the legacy of a trauma history. This principle applies to unlearning the maladaptive beliefs that are produced by any childhood scenario, traumatic or otherwise.

Finally, I want to stress the critical role of interpretation in those instances in which it is not a straightforward matter to pass the patient's tests. This consideration applies in instances in which the tests express a complicated and conflictual unconscious belief that puts the therapist in the position of being antitherapeutic no matter what stance is taken. For example, in a very common situation that too few of us are prepared for in our graduate training, a borderline and/or traumatized woman asks a therapist for a hug. The patient may be trying to disconfirm the pathogenic belief that caregivers are repelled by her. But simultaneously, she may be trying to disconfirm an equally powerful conviction that authorities will exploit her neediness for their own sensual and narcissistic gratification. Consequently, the therapist feels panicky, thinking, "It will hurt her feelings terribly if I don't hug her, because it will reinforce her conviction that she is disgusting. But if I do hug her, she will be terrified that I am taking advantage of her and cannot be trusted to maintain appropriate boundaries."

Thus, there is not a simple way to pass this test. But there is a complex one: The therapist can explain to the client that he or she feels in a terrible bind, that either hugging or not hugging her may be hurtful, and then go on to talk about the underlying beliefs that the therapist sees as at war in the patient's expression of the need for an embrace. The patient may not be happy to receive such an explanation, but it does skirt the Scylla of outright rejection and the Charybdis of seduction. And, ultimately, it can be assimilated to the client's benefit, once she works through the anger that her needs as immediately perceived have been frustrated. I would go so far as to say that every time a therapist feels in this kind of helpless dilemma (the "Omigod, whatever I do is wrong" phenomenon), it makes sense to look for an underlying pathogenic belief system in which two sides of a conflict are expressing themselves and needing the therapist's interpretative articulation. Sampson and Weiss would probably say that, in such instances, the interpretation *is* the passing of the test.

SUMMARY

In this chapter, I have explored the therapist's evaluation of the patient's conscious and unconscious cognitive world. I have briefly reviewed some psychoanalytic ideas about maladaptive unconscious beliefs, related them to cognitive-behavioral and family therapy insights about the role of unexamined assumptions in individuals and systems, and commented about my hopes for a rapprochement between analytic sensibilities on this issue and those of contemporary cognitive science. I have stressed the intractability of pathogenic beliefs, based on their having solved vital problems for each person in childhood, and I have particularly emphasized the importance of the therapist's accuracy in identifying the specific cognitions that operate pathogenically in individual patients. In discussing how to infer a person's problematic beliefs during an initial interview, I have counseled the reader to reflect on the interviewee's general comments about life, description of his or her upbringing, repetitive behavior, and transference reactions.

In considering the clinical implications of correctly deducing a patient's pathogenic ideas, I have talked mainly about the work of the San Francisco Psychotherapy Research Group, especially about their emphasis on patients' plans for recovery via devising tests by which the therapist will either confirm or disconfirm their preexisting unconscious convictions. I have given examples of how a therapist can pass both transference tests and passive-into-active tests, and then commented on the importance of also helping the patient to understand the beliefs behind the tests, their early origins, their functionality in childhood, and their dysfunctionality in the client's current life. I have given special attention to complex and conflictual pathogenic beliefs and the challenges they pose to a therapist's creativity.

Concluding Comments

THE shift from getting a general sense of a person to conceptualizing that individual's central dynamics is not always easily made. Case formulation goes way beyond nosology. Not only is it more ambitious than descriptive psychiatric taxonomy, the tradition exemplified in the DSM, but it also attempts more than the in-depth psychoanalytic character assessment I described in *Psychoanalytic Diagnosis* (cf. Westen, 1998). Formulating a case is a subjective, speculative, individualized, and comprehensive process. It requires getting a sense of someone's idiosyncratic inner life, feeling one's way into different aspects of that person's private world, trying to understand how it is to live life in that person's skin. One reason I have cautioned against going into a clinical interview trying to address head-on the questions I have covered in this book is that one needs to tolerate some disorganization and ambiguity in the process of letting the patient's psychology make an impact on one's own.

In the last few chapters, I have emphasized the treatment implications of different answers to central questions that therapists pose internally while listening to the story of any given client. I now return to the topic of the process, the art, of formulating a case. I hope it is helpful to the reader both in thinking about clients and in writing case reports in which a dynamic formulation is expected. It is valuable to set aside a little time after a intake interview to observe one's own subjective reactions to the client. What internal visual images have accompanied the interview? For example, does the person strike you as a porcelain doll, a mischievous little boy, a deer in the headlights, a volcano about to erupt? What feelings has the client evoked in you, and how strong are they? Is your body tense? If so, where? What parts of the person's experience seem strikingly like your own, and what parts are more alien? Does the patient remind you of anyone? Is there a song going through your head, and if so, what are the lyrics? What are your anxieties about working with this person? How would you put words to the combination of images and feelings you have accessed? Let your intuition have free rein for a while.

To access the degree of empathy necessary for effective therapy, it is important to appreciate any similarity between yourself and a client. Although all of us have been warned by supervisors not to overidentify with our patients, I feel strongly that overidentification is a much less serious failing than underidentification. Overidentification is forgivable by the client and correctable by the therapist. Because it represents an egalitarian position ("You and I have a lot in common"), it is not off-putting or humiliating. Beyond this, it seems to me incontrovertible that one cannot generate a meaningful sense of a person's subjective world without calling on one's own emotional history. All great actors know this: In order to give life to a role, one must find in the character something that resonates with a part of one's self. If a patient senses you are not able to feel a basic human kinship and similarity, he or she will despair of feeling uncritically understood.

Two people may have identical diagnoses and yet inhabit substantially different internal worlds. To illustrate this assertion, and in the process to demonstrate how to express a dynamic formulation, let me compare and contrast two women I will call Amanda and Beth, both of whom completed an analysis of several years' duration with me. Both came to me with depressive symptoms; each had a diagnosable dysthymic disorder and a depressively organized personality. Amanda and Beth were both health care professionals (a nurse and a physical therapist, respectively), and each brought considerable psychological sophistication to her work. Both were lesbians who had been "out" for many years. At the time each woman entered analysis with me, she had been living for several years with a partner with whom she was committed and content. Both came from families troubled by alcoholism. Amanda and Beth were alike also in being in the neurotic/healthy range of character structure, though each client's self-doubt expressed itself as a fear that as I knew her better, I would learn she was in some fundamental sense borderline. Both had had prior therapy and had chosen psychoanalytic treatment not only for its potential to relieve depressive symptoms but also for its promise to promote personal and professional growth.

There the similarities end. Amanda was from an Anglo-Saxon

Protestant, working-class family that moved several times during her childhood. Beth's family was Italian Catholic, upper-middle-class, and rooted in one community throughout her growing-up years. Amanda had a more bidirectional sexuality; she had been unhappily married to a man for several years before finding satisfaction with a woman. Beth had been attracted exclusively to females since puberty, if not before. In terms of temperament and unchangeable qualities, Amanda seems to have always been a very active and intense child. She and I invited her mother to a session late in her therapy and heard numerous stories about Amanda's energetic, demanding nature. Beth had grown up with comments about her quiet, self-contained temperament; her parents were proud of her capacity to amuse herself alone, even before age one.

Maturationally, both women got off to a good start, with what Winnicott would have called "good-enough" mothering in the first year. But Amanda's mother suffered a fairly severe depression after bearing a son when Amanda was fifteen months old. Her father's adaptation to parenthood, especially once his wife became ill, was a combination of avoidance, explosivity, and drink. Although Beth's mother soon became a problem drinker, in Beth's preschool years she seems to have been relatively abstemious and adequately protective. Beth's father was distant, intellectualized, and responsive to his daughter only when he was showing her off to others. He frequently insisted that she dress up and put on piano or dance performances or show off her skill at spelling. Both women had suffered sexual mistreatment as young children, Amanda from a grandfather who had also molested her mother, and Beth from a brother four years older. Amanda had fought off the abuse, which she experienced as hostile and intrusive, while Beth had been guiltily involved with her brother from age five to thirteen, when she began to menstruate and fear pregnancy.

Amanda and Beth had oedipal rather than preoedipal psychologies: Their subjectivities were not dominated by wishes either to fuse with or to struggle against a maternal object. They were able to see other people as complex combinations of positive and negative features, to feel desire for another whole person who is a separate and not unduly idealized object, to compete for affection, to identify with positive aspects of early love objects. Each woman had the homosexual version of the oedipal triangle; her same-sex parent had been her object of desire, and she had felt competitive with her father for her mother's love and attention. Being essentially dysthymic, both women used the central defenses of depressive people: They internalized negativity, projected their good attributes on to others, and tried to compensate for a self-esteem deficit by being generous and caretaking. Sensitive to loss and criticism and chronically susceptible to self-blame, they attributed their successes to good luck or to help from others and their failures to their personal defects. They differed, however, in some features of their defensive organization. Amanda saw negative qualities in others and then attacked them; Beth handled conflict with efforts to distance from problematic people. Amanda was hyperalert to my shortcomings and pushed to understand and process any empathic rupture between us. Beth was in treatment three years before she allowed herself to notice any instance in which I had hurt her feelings. Both women feared dependency; Amanda expressed it with a kind of "I can do it myself" bravado, and Beth tended to withdraw in intimate relationships.

Their affect patterns also differed. Amanda was more subject to irritation and anger, while Beth experienced a pervasive self-criticism and diffuse sorrow. Amanda tended to use anger to ward off feelings of grief, whereas Beth used sadness in the service of denying hostility. Amanda was frequently anxious, but Beth experienced anxiety only when called upon to do something she thought of as a "performance." Amanda was more subject to states of euphoria and elation; a quiet contentment was Beth's version of a good mood. Amanda's affective life was dominated by shame, expressing itself in the fear of exposure and humiliation, in contrast to Beth's tendency to feel guilt, inner badness, and a sense of culpability.

In terms of their respective identifications, Amanda was more stubbornly counteridentified than Beth. She shunned behavior that reminded her of her mother, and she bristled at any comments I made to the effect that she had nonetheless identified with her in certain ways. She had a positive identification with her father's role outside the family—he was a scientist with an admirable capacity for curiosity and wonder—but she mostly saw him as "other," as dangerous, as self-destructive and prone to violence. She found other authorities to emulate as she grew up and felt pleasure in differentiating herself from both parents. There was some evidence of her unconscious identification with her father, perhaps related to the fact that he had been the parent with more power. Beth, on the other hand, was positively identified with her mother, whom she initially described as "saintly." She was ambivalently identified with her father, whose intellect she admired, but whose self-absorption she blamed for her mother's drinking. Her comments in the intake interview suggested that she fended off negative perceptions of both parents, though she was able to express some resentment of the way her otherwise negligent father had wanted to display her when it suited his purposes. When I asked where her parents were during the many years when she and her brother were involved incestuously, she seemed to feel surprised by my implication that some supervision should have been going on.

The relational patterns of these two women were markedly divergent. Amanda tended to expect abuse by people in power and to behave provocatively when she feared that some kind of mistreatment was imminent. She had strained relations with hospital authorities and was perceived by some of her colleagues and superiors as prickly or oversensitive. In her professional role, she kept clear boundaries and was good at setting limits with patients, who found her concerned and reliable but not particularly warm and fuzzy. Beth tended to see authorities not as powerful and threatening, but as weak and ineffective. She tried to be invisible to them whenever possible, and she rarely questioned anything they asked her to do. She seldom took on roles that called attention to herself and was happiest when no one was interfering with her efficient way of carrying out her duties. With her patients, she was generous and self-effacing. Both women were fascinated by people and their idiosyncrasies, but whereas Amanda tended to use her analysis to figure out the psychologies of her supervisors, Beth usually discussed her patients.

Amanda's earliest dreams and fantasies in therapy portrayed me as hurt and vulnerable, and needing rescue from her. Over time, she developed a clear and somewhat erotized transference, and in the final stages of her analysis, she found in me the abusive father from whom she had to protect herself. My countertransference with Amanda was usually intense, sometimes irritably so and at other times more aroused, either sexually or in terms of general affect. Beth's experience of me was for a long time inscrutable. She did not like to discuss her feelings about me and seemed to feel interrupted and distracted when I would investigate this area. Eventually, she noticed that she assumed I was not particularly interested in her. A compelling fantasy emerged that I cared about her only insofar as her improvement in treatment would make me look good. With Beth my countertransference was consistently warm and steady, but not very driving. I sometimes felt bored during her sessions, and more than once I had to fight off sleep. I felt a deep affection for both women, but it expressed itself as more urgent and reactive with Amanda and more low-key with Beth.

Both women reacted strongly to separations, Amanda with anger, and Beth with preemptive withdrawal (before a break in treatment, she would become vague and elusive, and then miss our final appointment). In their intimate lives, they were also different: Amanda tended to initiate sexual relations with her partner and to enjoy sex frequently, something she talked about readily despite a normal amount of self-consciousness in disclosing private details of her life. Beth and her partner seldom made love and tended to do so only at the initiative of her lover. Beth could not bear to talk about her sexual experiences until the last year of her analysis. Amanda liked vigorous physical activity and sought out opportunities to do things in groups, while Beth's idea of a good time was to go fishing alone or curl up with a good book.

Each woman derived significant self-esteem from her professional role, from her attachments, from her general sensitivity to others, and from her commitment to pursuing personal growth and emotional maturity. Both felt considerable pride in having traversed the difficult coming-out process and in representing a proactive, positive lesbian identity. But Amanda's self-esteem was also reactive to the issue of whether anyone was "getting over" on her or using her. She had a deep need to speak truth to power. Her mood would plummet if she felt she had been manipulated or outsmarted. These issues were not salient to Beth, who put more emphasis on staying out of trouble. She would go through depressive reactions when she felt isolated or neglected, or when someone she cared about withdrew from her.

In terms of their respective pathogenic beliefs, although they both tended to have explanatory sets emphasizing their own badness and inadequacy, the content of that general percept differed between them. Amanda's central depressive convictions seemed to be as follows:

> "I'm too much for people. I'm too demanding and difficult. I wore my mother out, and my father saw my badness and punished me for it. Although I deserve his abuse, I have to do whatever I can to anticipate it and protect myself. I was not good enough to heal my mother, and ultimately I'm going to be found out and rejected. Anyone who knows me well will see how bad I am. If I confront others with their badness first, maybe I'll distract them from my own defects."

Beth's seemed to be more or less as follows:

> "I failed to help my mother with her sadness and her alcoholism. I can please my father by showing off for him, but when I do this, I feel unseen and used. The further I stay away from both parents, the less I will have to face the pain of my inability to get them to behave differently. I'll go through the motions of being a good girl,

but I'll create my own private world. I am bad for having the needs that have made sex with my brother attractive. The physical contact comforts me, but it also makes me feel sinful and alien to the rest of the human race. If I can hide effectively enough, no one will see how ineffectual and depraved I am."

The atmosphere in treatment of each of these women was quite different, even though the therapy of both could be properly depicted as classical psychoanalysis. After the initial interview with Amanda, I found myself very stimulated and excited about the prospect of a long, in-depth exploration. I also noticed some fears that I would disappoint her. Because of her emotional intensity, her penetrating way of looking at me, and the incisiveness of her initial questions, I had a subtle sense of being on trial. It was not hard to imagine that any authorities with a susceptibility to anxieties about their role would find Amanda intimidating. And, in fact, periodically during the treatment, I had to cope with the sense that I had failed her or hurt her, as she relived in the transference many of the actively hurtful things that had happened to her.

With Beth, I felt more serenely reflective and less on the defensive. I noticed a melody going through my head during her intake session— Carly Simon's despairing "That's the Way I Always Heard It Should Be." I found myself expecting that the key ingredients to her treatment would be the opportunity to access her anger and her energy in relationship with a person who would neither ignore her nor exploit her. In contrast to the need for relief I sometimes felt in the heat of an exchange with Amanda, I felt a kind of stimulus–hunger when working with Beth. I wanted to penetrate the wall of her withdrawal, to shake her up, to enliven her.

There follows a short case formulation about each woman, in which appear several of the topics I have covered in this book. I have linked them etiologically to each client's personal history and functionally to the specific goals each analysand articulated for her therapy, above and beyond conquering her depressive symptoms. The length of each statement is about what would be expected in the "dynamic formulation" section of a thorough case report. Here is a short version of some of Amanda's dynamics:

"Amanda has a depressive psychology deriving ultimately from a problematic fit between her own needs as an energetic and intense child and her mother's depressed state, starting when she was fifteen months old. Her father, temperamentally unable to compensate emotionally for her mother's withdrawal, seems to have related to her with irritation, hostility, and physical abuse. Her displacement by a favored son reinforced her sense that there was not enough love available for her. She seems to have concluded that she did not deserve to be cared for and that males will get whatever resources exist in a system, while women will be mistreated. This percept inclines her to feel like a magnet for abuse when she experiences herself as soft or feminine. She defends against sadness, which feels passive to her, with anger and activity. One of her goals for therapy is to access the more vulnerable side of herself, the pursuit of which can be expected to activate anxiety about her safety. The anger that accompanied her early deprivation seems to express itself in a readiness to confront authorities, whom she sees as unresponsive and abusive, like her father, or self-absorbed and ineffectual, like her mother. Consequently, another of her goals is to become less provocative toward those with power over her."

Here is a summary of some of Beth's central psychological issues:

"Beth has a depressive psychology that seems to derive from feeling that she could never help her alcoholic mother, and that if she did not cooperate with her narcissistic father's need to show her off, she would not get any attention at all. She tries to stay at arm's length from people lest their neediness absorb her or their exploitation make her feel like a soulless, manipulable object. A temperamentally sensitive, self-reliant child, she saw that neither parent had the emotional resources to invest in her deeply. She turned to her also neglected older brother for comfort and stimulation, which became sexualized. Beth suffers considerable self-hatred for her complicity with incest. She defends against strong feelings, both anger and passionate attachment, with feelings of sadness and self-criticism. She has come to therapy hoping to become more present and related, more sensual, less afraid of ordinary dependent wishes, and less suffused with guilt and the wish to withdraw."

Both women did very well in analysis. They remain appreciative of the difference it has made in their lives. Each was able to attain the treatment goals she had set, as well as other accomplishments not initially articulated (becoming more physically fit, managing money better, becoming less anxious about public speaking, using time more efficiently, having fewer colds and other illnesses, having better judgment about friends, feeling an increase in inner serenity, and developing new outlets for creativity, among others). But beyond their common need for an interested, nonjudgmental, nonintrusive therapist, their treatment requisites were quite different. Amanda needed me to withstand provocation and confrontation, and to help her work through hostile states of mind to the pain behind them; she responded well to my having solid boundaries and conveying a sense of confidence and power. Beth needed me to understand her pain, to be emotionally invested in who she really was, to insist that she let me into her private world of self-condemnation and detachment.

I hope these examples illustrate the ways one can assemble the information one gets in an intake interview. The whole is always psychologically bigger than the sum of the parts. Different practitioners will emphasize different aspects of a dynamic formulation, just as different clinicians will take things up in a different order during psychotherapy. Any therapeutic dyad creates its own two-person dynamic and interpersonal space, in which both parties struggle to make sense of what happens between them.

SOME FINAL ADVICE

Let me conclude with a few generalizations for the reader. Do not expect to have a handle on someone's psychology after a single visit. By the time you have been with a new person for a hour or so, however, you should be able to make some conjectures about his or her fixed attributes, developmental challenges, defenses, affects, identifications, relational patterns, self-esteem requirements, and pathogenic beliefs. Reflect on your hypotheses, think about the evidence for them, and consider their implications for treatment. When you have been taught a technique that makes no sense with a given individual in light of your understanding of the preceding areas, avoid that approach. A generally helpful clinical practice can, if applied to the wrong person, impose a hurtful misunderstanding of what is unchangeable, or violate developmental requisites, or fortify maladaptive defenses, or suppress authentic feelings, or affront basic identifications, or reinforce self-defeating interpersonal styles, or injure self-esteem, or reinforce pathogenic beliefs.

As I suggested in Chapter Six, a time-tested corrective to the limitations of any treater's individual subjectivity is the opportunity to present patients in depth to colleagues. In a group setting, elements of formulation that the treating practitioner has missed will be picked up by someone else. Most conscientious therapists I know go regularly to peer supervision groups or case seminars or consultation groups led by senior colleagues. These meetings give the presenting clinician a safe place to explore the affective dimension of his or her responses to clients and allow for a rich exchange of reactions to the clinical material (see Robbins, 1988). Because every patient who is discussed offers something new, thereby expanding the expertise of the participating therapists, such associations tend to have a long lifespan. Some of the professional groups in my area have been functioning continuously for over thirty years. One never gets too experienced to learn something eye-opening about oneself and one's clients.

Finally, keep letting your patients know that your curiosity about their actual feelings, fantasies, beliefs, and actions is greater than your need to get validation for your own formulations—or Freud's, or Kohut's, or Kernberg's, or Mitchell's, or those of anyone else you are tempted to idealize. Truths are usually surprising and often painful, to the client if not to the therapist whose narcissism bridles at admitting prior ignorance and misunderstanding. Yet most people are eventually willing to consider that what is true may be what is therapeutic. The commitment to discern and acknowledge unpleasant truths about human nature is perhaps the most consistently admirable feature of the checkered history of the psychoanalytic movement. And in a time when traditional psychotherapy is under enormous pressure to abandon the wisdom of decades of thoughtful and compassionate practitioners—not to mention the experience of the countless clients they have helped—the will to speak the truth is the strongest protection we have.

《〇》

Sample Contract

Welcome to my practice. There follows some essential information about psychotherapy. Please read and sign at the bottom to indicate that you have reviewed this information.

Length and frequency of treatment: Psychotherapy typically involves regular sessions, usually forty-five minutes in length. Duration and frequency vary depending on the nature of your problem and your individual needs.

Confidentiality: Information you share with me will be kept strictly confidential and will not be disclosed without your written consent. By law, however, confidentiality is not guaranteed in life-threatening situations involving yourself or others, or in situations in which children are put at risk (such as by sexual or physical abuse or neglect). If I need to discuss your treatment with a colleague, I will take pains to disguise identifying information, including using a pseudonym.

Fee policies: My fee for an individual therapy session is $ _____. If you need to cancel an appointment, please tell me at least twenty-four hours ahead of time; otherwise, I may charge you for the missed session. Please be aware that insurance carriers will not cover cancellation charges.

If you carry mental health insurance coverage, I will bill your carrier and assist with insurance reimbursement. In many circumstances, the insurance carrier limits the fee charged for the session. You will not be charged for the difference between my ordinary fee and the cap placed by insurance. Any copayment necessary should be made at the time of the office visit. Unless we make another explicit arrangement, you are responsible for filing insurance claims.

Phone and emergency contact: If you need to contact me by phone, do not hesitate. When I am not available, my answering machine will take a message. I am usually able to return calls within the day. You will not be charged for phone calls unless we have a scheduled conversation of an information-exchanging or problem-solving nature that lasts more than ten minutes. Phone sessions will be indicated as such on receipts and are not generally reimbursed by insurance. If you cannot reach me in an emergency, you can find help at the Emergency Services number of the local hospital: _____ (phone number).

Physician contact: Physical and psychological symptoms often interact. I encourage you to seek medical consultation if warranted. In addition, medication may sometimes be helpful for psychological problems. When appropriate, I will arrange a referral for medication evaluation.

Freedom to withdraw: You have the right to end therapy at any time. If you wish, I will give you the names of other qualified psychotherapists.

Informed consent: I have read and understood the preceding statements. I have had an opportunity to ask questions about them, and I agree to enter a professional psychotherapy relationship with _____ _____ (practitioner's name).

Patient _____ Date _____

References

Abraham, K. (1911). Notes on the psycho-analytical investigation and treatment of manic–depressive insanity and allied conditions. In J. D. Sutherland (Ed.), *Selected papers of Karl Abraham* (pp. 137–156). London: Hogarth Press, 1968.

Acosta, F. X. (1984). *Psychotherapy with Mexican-Americans: Clinical and empirical gains.* In J. L. Martinez, Jr. & R. H. Mendoza (Eds.), *Chicano psychology* (2nd ed., pp. 163–189). New York: Academic Press.

Adler, A. (1927). *Understanding human nature.* Garden City, NY: Garden City Publishing.

Adler, A. (1931). *What life should mean to you.* Boston: Little, Brown.

Ainsworth, M. D. S., Blehar, M. C., Waters, E., & Wall, S. (1978). *Patterns of attachment: A psychological study of the strange situation.* Hillsdale, NJ: Erlbaum.

Akhtar, S. (1992). *Broken structures: Severe personality disorders and their treatment.* Northvale, NJ: Aronson.

Alexander, F. (1956). *Psychoanalysis and psychotherapy: Developments in theory, technique and training.* New York: Norton.

Allport, G. W. (1961). *Pattern and growth in personality.* New York: Holt, Rinehart & Winston.

Altman, N. (1995). *The analyst in the inner city: Race, class, and culture through a psychoanalytic lens.* Hillsdale, NJ: Analytic Press.

American Psychiatric Association. (1968). *Diagnostic and statistical manual of mental disorders* (2nd ed). Washington, DC: Author.

American Psychiatric Association. (1980). *Diagnostic and statistical manual of mental disorders* (3rd ed.). Washington, DC: Author.

American Psychiatric Association. (1987). *Diagnostic and statistical manual of mental disorders* (3rd ed., rev.). Washington, DC: Author.

American Psychiatric Association. (1994). *Diagnostic and statistical manual of mental disorders* (4th ed.). Washington, DC: Author.

Aries, P. (1962). *Centuries of childhood.* New York: Knopf.

Arkowitz, H., & Messer, S. B. (1984). *Psychoanalytic therapy and behavior therapy: Is integration possible?* New York: Plenum.

Aron, L. (1990). One-person and two-person psychologies and the method of psychoanalysis. *Psychoanalytic Psychology, 7,* 475–485.

Aron, L. (1996). *A meeting of minds: Mutuality in psychoanalysis.* Hillsdale, NJ: Analytic Press.

Atwood, G. E., & Stolorow, R. D. (1984). *Structures of subjectivity: Explorations in psychoanalytic phenomenology.* Hillsdale, NJ: Analytic Press.

Bach, S. (1985). *Narcissistic states and the therapeutic process.* New York: Aronson.

Balint, M. (1960). Primary narcissism and primary love. *Psychoanalytic Quarterly, 29,* 6–43.

Balint, M. (1968). *The basic fault: Therapeutic aspects of regression.* London: Tavistock.

Barlow, D. (1998, August 14). [Untitled paper.] In M. Patterson (Chair), *Future of the scientist-practitioner.* Symposium conducted at the 106th annual meeting of the American Psychological Association, San Francisco, CA.

Barron, J. W. (Ed.). (1998). *Making diagnosis meaningful: Enhancing evaluation and treatment of psychological disorders.* Washington, DC: American Psychological Association.

Barron, J. W., Eagle, M. N., & Wolitzky, D. L. (Eds.). (1992). *Interface of psychoanalysis and psychology.* Washington, DC: American Psychological Association.

Barron, J. W., & Sands, H. (1996). *Impact of managed care on psychodynamic treatment.* Madison, CT: International Universities Press.

Beebe, B., & Lachmann, F. M. (1988). The contribution of mother–infant mutual influence to the origins of self- and object relationships. *Psychoanalytic Psychology, 5,* 305–337.

Bellak, L. (1954). *The Thematic Apperception Test and the Children's Apperception Test in clinical use.* New York: Grune & Stratton.

Bellak, L., & Small, L. (1965). *Emergency psychotherapy and brief psychotherapy.* New York: Grune & Stratton.

Benjamin, J. (1988). *The bonds of love: Psychoanalysis, feminism, and the problem of domination.* New York: Pantheon.

Benjamin, L. S. (1993). *Interpersonal diagnosis and treatment of personality disorders.* New York: Guilford Press.

Beres, D. (1958). Vicissitudes of superego formation and superego precursors in childhood. *Psychoanalytic Study of the Child, 13,* 324–335.

Bergmann, M. S. (1987). *The anatomy of loving: The story of man's quest to know what love is.* New York: Columbia University Press.

Berliner, B. (1958). The role of object relations in moral masochism. *Psychoanalytic Quarterly, 27,* 38–56.

Berne, E. (1974). Transactional analysis. In H. Greenwald (Ed.), *Active psychotherapy* (pp. 119–129). New York: Aronson.

Bernstein, D. (1993). *Female identity conflict in clinical practice* (N. Freedman & B. Distler, Eds.). Northvale, NJ: Aronson.

Bettelheim, B. (1954). *Symbolic wounds: Puberty rites and the envious male.* Glencoe, IL: Free Press.

Bettelheim, B. (1960). *The informed heart: Autonomy in a mass age.* Glencoe, IL: Free Press.

Blanck, G., & Blanck, R. (1974). *Ego psychology: Theory and practice.* New York: Columbia University Press.

Blanck, G., & Blanck, R. (1979). *Ego psychology II: Psychoanalytic developmental psychology.* New York: Columbia University Press.

Blanck, R., & Blanck, G. (1986). *Beyond ego psychology: Developmental object relations theory.* New York: Columbia University Press.

Blatt, S., & Levy, K. (1998). A psychodynamic approach to the diagnosis of psychopathology. In J. W. Barron (Ed.), *Making diagnosis meaningful: Enhancing evaluation and treatment of psychological disorders* (pp. 73–110). Washington, DC: American Psychological Association.

Blechner, M. J. (Ed.). (1997). *Hope and mortality: Psychodynamic approaches to AIDS and HIV.* Mahwah, NJ: Analytic Press.

Blos, P. (1962). *On adolescence: A psychoanalytic interpretation.* New York: Free Press of Glencoe.

Bollas, C. (1987). *The shadow of the object: Psychoanalysis of the unthought known.* New York: Columbia University Press.

Bornstein, R. F. (1993). Parental representations and psychopathology: A critical review of the empirical literature. In J. M. Masling & R. F. Bornstein (Eds.), *Psychoanalytic perspectives on psychopathology* (pp. 1–41). Washington, DC: American Psychological Association.

Bornstein, R. F., & Masling, J. M. (Eds.). (1998). *Empirical perspectives on the psychoanalytic unconscious.* Washington, DC: American Psychological Association.

Bowlby, J. (1969). *Attachment and loss: Vol. 1. Attachment.* New York: Basic Books.

Bowlby, J. (1973). *Attachment and loss: Vol. 2. Separation: Anxiety and anger.* New York: Basic Books.

Bowlby, J. (1980). *Attachment and loss: Vol. 3. Loss: Sadness and depression.* New York: Basic Books.

Boyd-Franklin, N. (1989). *Black families in therapy: A multisystems approach.* New York: Guilford Press.

Brazelton, T. B., Koslowski, B., & Main, M. (1974). The origins of reciprocity: The early mother–infant interaction. In M. Lewis & L. Rosenblum (Eds.), *The effect of the infant on its caregiver* (pp. 49–76). New York: Wiley.

Brazelton, T. B., Yogman, M., Als, H., & Tronick, E. (1979). Joint regulation of neonate–parent behavior. In E. Tronick (Ed.), *Social interchange in infancy* (pp. 7–22). Baltimore: University Park Press.

Bretherton, I. (1998, October 2). *From interaffectivity and attunement to shared meanings: An attachment perspective on individual differences.* Paper presented at a conference on "Mutual Understanding," University of Crete, Rethymnon, Crete, Greece.

Bridges, K. M. B. (1931). *The social and emotional development of the pre-school child.* London: Kegan Paul.

Brooke, R. (1994). Assessment for psychotherapy: Clinical indicators of self cohesion and self pathology. *British Journal of Psychotherapy, 10,* 317–330.

Bucci, W. (1985). Dual coding: A cognitive model for psychoanalytic research. *Journal of the American Psychoanalytic Association, 33,* 571–607.

Bucci, W. (1997). *Psychoanalysis and cognitive science: A multiple code theory.* New York: Guilford Press.

Bursten, B. (1973). *The manipulator: A psychoanalytic view.* New Haven, CT: Yale University Press.

Butler, D. A. (1998). *"Unsinkable": The full story of RMS Titanic*. Mechanicsburg, PA: Stackpole Books.

Calef, V., & Weinshel, E. (1981). Some clinical consequences of introjection: Gaslighting. *Psychoanalytic Quarterly, 50*, 44–66.

Callahan, R. J., & Callahan, J. (1996). *Thought field therapy and trauma: Treatment and theory*. Indian Wells, CA: Authors.

Cardinal, M. (1983). *The words to say it*. Cambridge, MA: VanVactor & Goodheart.

Carlson, R. (1986). After analysis: A study of transference dreams following treatment. *Journal of Consulting and Clinical Psychology, 54*, 246–252.

Carotenuto, A. (Ed.). (1983). *A secret symmetry: Sabina Spielrein between Jung and Freud* (rev. ed.). New York: Pantheon.

Chessick, R. D. (1983). *How psychotherapy heals: The process of intensive psychotherapy*. Northvale, NJ: Aronson.

Clark, L. A., Watson, D., & Reynolds, S. (1995). Diagnosis and classification of psychopathology: Challenges to the current system and future directions. In J. T. Spence, J. M. Darley, & D. J. Foss (Eds.), *Annual review of psychology* (Vol. 46, pp. 121–153). Palo Alto, CA: Annual Reviews.

Cleckley, H. (1941). *The mask of sanity: An attempt to clarify some issues about the so-called psychopathic personality*. St. Louis: Mosby.

Comas-Díaz, L., & Greene, B. (Eds.). (1994). *Women of color: Integrating ethnic and gender identities in psychotherapy*. New York: Guilford Press.

Dahl, H. (1988). Frames of mind. In H. Dahl, H. Kachele, & H. Thomae (Eds.), *Psychoanalytic process research strategies* (pp. 51–66). New York: Springer-Verlag.

Davies, J. M. (1994). Love in the afternoon: A relational reconsideration of desire and dread in the countertransference. *Psychoanalytic Dialogues, 4*, 153–170.

Davies, J. M., & Frawley, M. G. (1993). *Treating the adult survivor of childhood sexual abuse: A psychoanalytic perspective*. New York: Basic Books.

Dennis, P. (1955). *Auntie Mame*. New York: Buccaneer Books, 1995.

Dowling, S., & Rothstein, A. (Eds.). (1989). *The significance of infant observational research for clinical work with children, adolescents and adults*. Madison, CT: International Universities Press.

Eissler, K. R. (1953). The effects of the structure of the ego on psychoanalytic technique. *Journal of the American Psychoanalytic Association, 1*, 104–143.

Ekman, P. (1971). Universals and cultural differences in facial expressions of emotion. In J. Cole (Ed.), *Nebraska symposium on motivation 1971* (pp. 207–283). Lincoln: University of Nebraska Press.

Ekman, P. (1980). *The face of man: Expressions of universal emotions in a New Guinea village*. New York: Garland STPM Press.

Elkind, S. N. (1992). *Resolving impasses in therapeutic relationships*. New York: Guilford Press.

Emde, R. N. (1990). Mobilizing fundamental modes of development: An essay on empathic availability. *Journal of the American Psychoanalytic Association, 38*, 881–914.

Emde, R. N. (1991). Positive emotions for psychoanalytic theory: Surprises from infancy research and new directions. *Journal of the American Psychoanalytic Association, 39*, 5–14.

Epstein, M. (1998). *Going to pieces without falling apart: A Buddhist perspective on wholeness (Lessons from meditation and psychotherapy)*. New York: Broadway Books.

Erikson, E. H. (1950). *Childhood and society*. New York: Norton.

Erikson, E. H. (1968). *Identity: Youth and crisis*. New York: Norton.

Erikson, E. H. (1997). *The life cycle completed*. New York: Norton.

Escalona, S. K. (1968). *The roots of individuality: Normal patterns of development in infancy*. Chicago: Aldine.

Etchegoyen, R. H. (1991). *The fundamentals of psychoanalytic technique*. London: Karnac Books.

Fairbairn, W. R. D. (1952). *An object-relations theory of the personality*. New York: Basic Books.

Fast, I. (1998). *Selving: A relational theory of self organization*. Hillsdale, NJ: Analytic Press.

Fenichel, O. (1941). *Problems of psychoanalytic technique*. Albany, NY: Psychoanalytic Quarterly.

Fenichel, O. (1945). *The psychoanalytic theory of neurosis*. New York: Norton.

Fisher, S., & Greenberg, R. P. (1985). *The scientific credibility of Freud's theories and therapy*. New York: Columbia University Press.

Fossum, M. A., & Mason, M. J. (1986). *Facing shame: Families in recovery*. New York: Norton.

Foster, R. P., Moskowitz, M., & Javier, R. A. (1996). *Reaching across boundaries of culture and class: Widening the scope of psychotherapy*. Northvale, NJ: Aronson.

Fraiberg, S. (Ed.). (1980). *Clinical studies in infant mental health: The first year of life*. New York: Basic Books.

Frank, E., Kupfer, D. J., & Siegel, L. R. (1995). Alliance not compliance: A philosophy of outpatient care. *Journal of Clinical Psychiatry, 56*, 11–17.

Frankl, V. E. (1969). *The doctor and the soul*. New York: Bantam.

Frawley-O'Dea, M. G. (1996, March 10). *Ah yes, I remember it well. Or do I?* Paper presented at the annual conference of the Institute for Psychoanalysis and Psychotherapy of New Jersey, Edison, NJ.

Freud, A. (1936). *The ego and the mechanisms of defense*. New York: International Universities Press, 1966.

Freud, A. (1970). The infantile neurosis: Genetic and dynamic considerations. In *The writings of Anna Freud* (Vol. 7, pp. 189–203). New York: International Universities Press.

Freud, S. (1894). The neuro-psychoses of defense. *Standard Edition, 3*, 45–61.

Freud, S. (1911). Formulations on the two principles of mental functioning. *Standard Edition, 12*, 218–226.

Freud, S. (1912). The dynamics of transference. *Standard Edition, 12*, 99–108.

Freud, S. (1913). On beginning the treatment (Further recommendations on the technique of psycho-analysis I). *Standard Edition, 12*, 123–144.

Freud, S. (1916). Some character-types met with in psycho-analytic work. *Standard Edition, 14*, 311–333.

Freud, S. (1917). Mourning and melancholia. *Standard Edition, 14*, 243–258.

Freud, S. (1920). Beyond the pleasure principle. *Standard Edition, 18*, 7–64.

Freud, S. (1921). Group psychology and the analysis of the ego. *Standard Edition, 18*, 105–110.

Freud, S. (1923). The ego and the id. *Standard Edition, 19*, 13–59.

Freud, S. (1926). The question of lay analysis: Conversations with an impartial person. *Standard Edition, 20,* 183–250.

Freud, S. (1933). The question of a Weltanschauung. *Standard Edition, 22,* 158–182.

Freud S. (1940). An outline of psycho-analysis. *Standard Edition, 23,* 141–207.

Freyd, J. J. (1996). *Betrayal trauma: The logic of forgetting childhood abuse.* Cambridge, MA: Harvard University Press.

Fromm, E. (1956). *The art of loving.* New York: Harper & Row.

Fromm-Reichmann, F. (1950). *Principles of intensive therapy.* Chicago: University of Chicago Press.

Frommer, M. S. (1995). Countertransference obscurity in the psychoanalytic treatment of homosexual patients. In T. Domenici & R. Lesser (Eds.), *Disorienting sexuality: Psychoanalytic reappraisals of sexual identities* (pp. 65–82). New York: Routledge.

Gabbard, G. O. (1994). Love and lust in the erotic transference. *Journal of the American Psychoanalytic Association, 42,* 385–403.

Gabbard, G. O. (1996). *Love and hate in the analytic setting.* Northvale, NJ: Aronson.

Gabbard, G. O., Lazar, S. G., Hornberger, J., & Spiegel, D. (1997). The economic impact of psychotherapy: A review. *American Journal of Psychiatry, 154,* 147–155.

Gabbard, G. O., & Lester, E. P. (1995). *Boundaries and boundary violations in psychoanalysis.* New York: Basic Books.

Gacano, C. B., & Meloy, J. R. (1994). *The Rorschach assessment of aggressive and psychopathic personalities.* Hillsdale, NJ: Erlbaum.

Galenson, E., & Roiphe, H. (1974). The emergence of genital awareness during the second year of life. In R. C. Friedman, R. M. Richart, & R. L. Van de Wides (Eds.), *Sex differences in behavior* (pp. 223–231). New York: Wiley.

Gallo, F. P. (1998). *Energy psychology: Explorations at the interface of energy, cognition, behavior, and health.* New York: CRC Press.

Gill, M. M. (1994). *Psychoanalysis in transition: A personal view.* Hillsdale, NJ: Analytic Press.

Gill, M. M., & Hoffman, I. (1982). A method for studying the analysis of aspects of the patient's experience of the relationship in psychoanalysis and psychotherapy. *Journal of the American Psychoanalytic Association, 30,* 137–167.

Gitlin, M. J. (1996). *The psychotherapist's guide to psychopharmacology* (2nd ed.). New York: Free Press.

Goldberg, F. H. (1998, April 25). *Coming late may not always be resistance: Psychoanalytic therapy with adults who have attention deficit disorder.* Paper presented at the spring meeting of the Division of Psychoanalysis, American Psychological Association, Boston, MA.

Goldfried, M. R., & Wolfe, B. E. (1996). Psychotherapy practice and research: Repairing a strained alliance. *American Psychologist, 51,* 1007–1016.

Goldstein, K. (1942). *Aftereffects of brain injuries in war, their evaluation and treatment; the application of psychologic methods in the clinic.* New York: Grune.

Goleman, D. (1995). *Emotional intelligence.* New York: Bantam.

Goodheart, C. D., & Lansing, M. H. (1997). *Treating people with chronic disease: A psychological guide.* Washington, DC: American Psychological Association.

Gottesman, I. I., & Shields, J. (1982). *Schizophrenia: The epigenetic puzzle*. Cambridge, UK: Cambridge University Press.

Greenberg, J. R., & Mitchell, S. A. (1983). *Object relations in psychoanalytic theory*. Cambridge, MA: Harvard University Press.

Greenberg, L. S., & Safran, J. D. (1987). *Emotion in psychotherapy: Affect, cognition, and the process of change*. New York: Guilford Press.

Greenson, R. R. (1967). *The technique and practice of psychoanalysis*. New York: International Universities Press.

Greenspan, S. I. (1981). *Clinical infant reports: Number 1. Psychopathology and adaptation in infancy and early childhood: Principles of clinical diagnosis and preventive intervention*. New York: International Universities Press.

Greenspan, S. I. (1989). *The development of the ego: Implications for personality theory, psychopathology, and the psychotherapeutic process*. Madison, CT: International Universities Press.

Greenspan, S. I. (1996). *The challenging child: Understanding, raising, and enjoying the five "difficult" types of children*. New York: Addison-Wesley.

Greenspan, S. I. (1997). *Developmentally based psychotherapy*. Madison, CT: International Universities Press.

Greenwald, H. (1958). *The call girl: A sociological and psychoanalytic study*. New York: Ballantine Books.

Grier, W., & Cobbs, P. (1968). *Black rage*. New York: Basic Books.

Guntrip, H. (1969). *Schizoid phenomena, object relations and the self*. New York: International Universities Press.

Haan, N. A. (1977). *Coping and defending*. San Francisco: Jossey-Bass.

Hall, G. S. (1904). *Adolescence: Its psychology and its relation to physiology, anthropology, sociology, sex, crime, religion, and education* (Vols. 1 and 2). New York: Appleton–Century–Crofts.

Hammer, E. (1990). *Reaching the affect: Style in the psychodynamic therapies*. New York: Aronson.

Hare, R. (1978). Electrodermal and cardiovascular correlates of psychopathy. In R. Hare & D. Schalling (Eds.), *Psychopathic behavior: Approaches to research* (pp. 107–143). Chichester, UK: Wiley.

Hare, R. (1991). *The Hare Psychopathy Checklist—Revised Manual*. Toronto: Multi-Health Systems.

Haugaard, J. J., & Reppucci, N. D. (1989). *The sexual abuse of children*. San Francisco: Jossey-Bass.

Henry, W. P., Schacht, T. E., & Strupp, H. H. (1986). Structural analysis of social behavior: Application to a study of interpersonal process in differential psychotherapeutic outcome. *Journal of Counseling and Clinical Psychology, 54*, 27–31.

Herman, J. L. (1992). *Trauma and recovery: The aftermath of violence—from domestic abuse to political terror*. New York: Basic Books.

Hertsgaard, L. (1995). Adrenocortical responses to the strange situation in infants with disorganized/disoriented attachment relationships. *Child Development, 66*, 1100–1106.

Hite, A. L. (1996). The diagnostic alliance. In D. Nathanson (Ed.), *Knowing feeling: Affect, script, and psychotherapy* (pp. 37–55). New York: Norton.

Horner, A. J. (1991). *Psychoanalytic object relations therapy*. Northvale, NJ: Aronson.

Horowitz, M. (1988). *Introduction to psychodynamics: A new synthesis*. New York: Basic Books.

Horowitz, M. (1991). Psychic structure and the process of change. In M. Horowitz (Ed.), *Hysterical personality style and the histrionic personality disorder* (pp. 193–261). Northvale, NJ: Aronson.

Howard, K. I., Moras, K., Brill, P. L., Martinovich, Z., & Lutz, W. (1996). Evaluation of psychotherapy: Efficacy, effectiveness, patient progress. *American Psychologist, 51,* 1059–1064.

Huang, M. Y., & Nunes, E. V. (1995). Substance induced persisting dementia and substance abuse persisting amnestic disorder. In G. O. Gabbard (Ed.), *Treatments of psychiatric disorders* (2nd ed., pp. 555–631). Washington, DC: American Psychiatric Press.

Hurvich, M. S. (1989). Traumatic moment, basic dangers and annihilation anxiety. *Psychoanalytic Psychology, 6,* 309–323.

Izard, C. E. (1971). *The face of emotion.* New York: Appleton–Century–Crofts.

Izard, C. E. (Ed.). (1979). *Emotions in personality and psychopathology.* New York: Plenum.

Jacobson, E. (1964). *The self and the object world.* New York: International Universities Press.

Jacobson, E. (1971). *Depression: Comparative studies of normal, neurotic, and psychotic conditions.* New York: International Universities Press.

Jahoda, M. (1958). *Current concepts of positive mental health.* New York: Basic Books.

Javier, R. A. (1990). The suitability of insight oriented therapy for the Hispanic poor. *American Journal of Psychoanalysis, 50,* 305–318.

Johnson, A. (1949). Sanctions for superego lacunae of adolescents. In K. R. Eissler (Ed.), *Searchlights on delinquency* (pp. 225–245). New York: International Universities Press.

Johnson, S. M. (1994). *Character styles.* New York: Norton.

Josephs, L. (1992). *Character structure and the organization of the self.* New York: Columbia University Press.

Josephs, L. (1995). *Balancing empathy and interpretation: Relational character analysis.* Northvale, NJ: Aronson.

Kagan, J. (1994). *Galen's prophecy: Temperament in human nature.* New York: Basic Books.

Kaplan, L. (1984). *Adolescence: The farewell to childhood.* New York: Simon & Schuster.

Karon, B. (1989). On the formation of delusions. *Psychoanalytic Psychology, 6,* 169–185.

Karon, B. (1998, August 16). *The tragedy of schizophrenia.* Paper presented at the 106th annual meeting of the American Psychological Association, San Francisco, CA.

Karon, B., & VandenBos, G. R. (1981). *Psychotherapy of schizophrenia: The treatment of choice.* New York: Aronson.

Kelly, K., & Ramundo, P. (1995). *You mean I'm not lazy, crazy, or stupid?!: A self-help book for adults with attention deficit disorder.* New York: Scribner.

Keniston, K. (1971). *Youth and dissent.* New York: Harcourt, Brace, Jovanovich.

Kernberg, O. F. (1975). *Borderline conditions and pathological narcissism.* New York: Aronson.

Kernberg, O. F. (1976). *Object relations theory and clinical psychoanalysis.* New York: Aronson.

Kernberg, O. F. (1984). *Severe personality disorders: Psychotherapeutic strategies.* New Haven, CT: Yale University Press.

Kernberg, O. F. (1992). *Aggression in personality disorders and perversions.* New Haven, CT: Yale University Press.

Kernberg, O. F. (1995). *Love relations: Normality and pathology.* New Haven, CT: Yale University Press.

Kernberg, O. F. (1997, December 6). *New developments in the diagnosis and treatment of narcissistic psychopathology.* Address given at Montefiore Medical Center, New York, NY.

Kernberg, O. F., Selzer, M. A., Koenigsberg, H. W., Carr, A. C., & Appelbaum, A. H. (1989). *Psychodynamic psychotherapy of borderline patients.* New York: Basic Books.

Kerr, J. (1993). *A most dangerous method: The story of Jung, Freud, and Sabina Spielrein.* New York: Vintage Books.

Kets de Vries, M. F. R. (1989). *Prisoners of leadership.* New York: Wiley.

Klein, M. (1946). Notes on some schizoid mechanisms. *International Journal of Psycho-Analysis, 27,* 99–110.

Klein, M. (1957). Envy and gratitude. In *Envy and gratitude and other works 1946–1963* (pp. 176–235). New York: Free Press, 1975.

Klerman, G. L., Weissman, M. M., Rounsaville, B. J., & Chevron, E. S. (1984). *Interpersonal psychotherapy of depression.* New York: Basic Books.

Kluft, R. P. (1991). Multiple personality disorder. In A. Tasman & S. M. Goldfinger (Eds.), *American Psychiatric Press review of psychiatry* (Vol. 10, pp. 161–188). Washington, DC: American Psychiatric Press.

Kobak, R., & Sceery, A. (1988). Attachment in late adolescence: Working models, affect regulation, and perception of self and others. *Child Development, 59,* 135–146.

Kohut, H. (1971). *The analysis of the self: A systematic approach to the psychoanalytic treatment of narcissistic personality disorders.* New York: International Universities Press.

Kohut, H. (1977). *The restoration of the self.* New York: International Universities Press.

Lachmann, F. M., & Lichtenberg, J. D. (1992). Model scenes: Implications for psychoanalytic treatment. *Journal of the American Psychoanalytic Association, 40,* 117–137.

Laing, R. D. (1965). *The divided self: An existential study in sanity and madness.* Baltimore: Penguin.

Lambert, M. J., & Bergin, A. E. (1994). The effectiveness of psychotherapy. In A. E. Bergin & S. L. Garfield (Eds.), *Handbook of psychotherapy and behavior change* (4th ed., pp. 467–508). New York: Wiley.

Lambert, M. J., Shapiro, D., & Bergin, A. E. (1986). The effectiveness of psychotherapy. In S. Garfield & A. Bergin (Eds.), *Handbook of psychotherapy and behavior change: An empirical analysis* (pp. 157–212). New York: Wiley.

Langs, R., & Stone, L. (1980). *The therapeutic experience and its setting: A clinical dialogue.* New York: Aronson.

Lasch, C. (1984). *The minimal self: Psychic survival in troubled times.* New York: Norton.

Lasky, E. (1984). Psychoanalysts' and psychotherapists' conflicts about setting fees. *Psychoanalytic Psychology, 1,* 289–300.

Laughlin, H. P. (1967). *The neuroses*. New York: Appleton–Century–Crofts.

LeDoux, J. E. (1995). Emotion: Clues from the brain. In J. T. Spence, J. M. Darley, & D. J. Foss (Eds.), *Annual review of psychology* (Vol. 46, pp. 209–235). Palo Alto, CA: Annual Reviews.

Lerner, H. G. (1985). *The dance of anger*. New York: Harper & Row.

Lerner, H. G. (1989). *The dance of intimacy*. New York: Harper & Row.

Lesser, R. D. (1995). Objectivity as masquerade. In T. Domenici & R. Lesser (Eds.), *Disorienting sexuality: Psychoanalytic reappraisals of sexual identities* (pp. 83–96). New York: Routledge.

Levenson, E. A. (1972). *The fallacy of understanding: An inquiry into the changing structure of psychoanalysis*. New York: Basic Books.

Levin, J. D. (1987). *Treatment of alcoholism and other addictions: A self psychology approach*. Northvale, NJ: Aronson.

Levinson, D. J., Darrow, C. N., Klein, E.B., Levinson, M. H., & McKee, B. (1978). *The seasons of a man's life*. New York: Knopf.

Lewis, D. O., Pincus, J. H., Bard, B., Richardson, E., Prichep, L. S., Feldman, M., & Yaeger, C. (1988). Neuropsychiatric, psychoeducational, and family characteristics of 14 juveniles condemned to death in he United States. *American Journal of Psychiatry, 145*, 584–589.

Lewis, D. O., Pincus, J. H., Feldman, M., Jackson, L., & Bard, B. (1986). Psychiatric, neurological, and psychoeducational characteristics of 15 death row inmates in the Unites States. *American Journal of Psychiatry, 143*, 838–845.

Lewis, H. B. (1971). *Shame and guilt in neurosis*. New York: International Universities Press.

Lichtenberg, J. D. (1983). *Psychoanalysis and infant research*. Hillside, NJ: Analytic Press.

Lichtenberg, J. D. (1989). *Psychoanalysis and motivation*. Hillsdale, NJ: Analytic Press.

Lichtenberg, J. D., Lachmann, F., & Fossage, J. (1992). *Self and motivational systems: Toward a theory of psychoanalytic technique*. Hillsdale, NJ: Analytic Press.

Lifton, R. J. (1968). *Death in life: Survivors of Hiroshima*. New York: Random House.

Lipsey, M. W., & Wilson, D. B. (1993). The efficacy of psychological, educational, and behavioral treatment: Confirmation from meta-analysis. *American Psychologist, 48*, 1181–1209.

Liss-Levinson, N. (1990). Money matters and the woman analyst: In a different voice. *Psychoanalytic Psychology, 7*, 119–130.

Loewald, H. W. (1957). On the therapeutic action of psychoanalysis. In *Papers on psycho-analysis* (pp. 221–256). New Haven, CT: Yale University Press, 1980.

Lovinger, R. J. (1984). *Working with religious issues in therapy*. New York: Aronson.

Luborsky, L., & Crits-Christoph, P. (1998). *Understanding transference: The core conflictual relationship theme* (2nd ed.). Washington, DC: American Psychological Association.

Luborsky, L., Singer, B., & Luborsky, L. (1975). Comparative studies of psychotherapies: Is it true that "Everyone has won and all must have prizes"? *Archives of General Psychiatry, 32*, 995–1008.

Lynd, H. M. (1958). *On shame and the search for identity.* New York: Harcourt, Brace & World.

MacEdo, S. (1991). *Liberal virtues: Citizenship, virtue, and community in liberal constitutionalism.* London: Oxford University Press.

MacKinnon, R. A., & Michels, R. (1971). *The psychiatric interview in clinical practice.* Philadelphia: Saunders.

Mahler, M. S. (1968). *On human symbiosis and the vicissitudes of individuation.* New York: International Universities Press.

Mahler, M. S. (1971). A study of the separation–individuation process and its possible application to borderline phenomena in the psychoanalytic situation. In *The selected papers of Margaret S. Mahler* (Vol. 2, pp. 169–187). New York: Aronson, 1979.

Mahler, M. S., Pine, F., & Bergman, A. (1975). *The psychological birth of the human infant.* New York: Basic Books.

Main, M., Kaplan, N., & Cassidy, J. (1985). Security in infancy, childhood, and adulthood: A move to the level of representation. *Monographs of the Society for Research in Child Development, 50*(1–2, Serial No. 209).

Main, M., & Solomon, J. (1986). Discovery of an insecure disorganized/disoriented attachment pattern: Procedures, findings and theoretical implications. In T. Brazelton & M. Yogman (Eds.), *Affective development in infancy* (pp. 95–124). Norwood, NJ: Ablex.

Malan, D.H. (1976). *The frontier of brief psychotherapy.* New York: Plenum.

Masling, J. M. (Ed.). (1983). *Empirical studies of psychoanalytic theories* (Vol. 1). Hillsdale, NJ: Analytic Press.

Masling, J. M. (Ed.). (1986). *Empirical studies of psychoanalytic theories* (Vol. 2). Hillsdale, NJ: Analytic Press.

Masling, J. M. (Ed.). (1990). *Empirical studies of psychoanalytic theories* (Vol. 3). Hillsdale, NJ: Analytic Press.

Masterson, J. F. (1976). *Psychotherapy of the borderline adult: A developmental approach.* New York: Brunner/Mazel.

McDougall, J. (1989). *Theaters of the body: A psychoanalytic approach to psychosomatic illness.* New York: Norton.

McFarlane, A. C., & van der Kolk, B. A. (1996). Trauma and its challenge to society. In B. A. van der Kolk, A. C. McFarlane, & L. Weisaeth (Eds.), *Traumatic stress: The effects of overwhelming experience on mind, body, and society* (pp. 24–46). New York: Guilford Press.

McGoldrick, M., Giordano, J., & Pearce, J. K. (Eds.). (1996). *Ethnicity and family therapy* (2nd ed.). New York: Guilford Press.

McGuire, W. (Ed.). (1974). *The Freud/Jung letters: The correspondence between Sigmund Freud and C. G. Jung* (R. Manheim & R. F. C. Hull, Trans.). Princeton, NJ: Princeton University Press.

McWilliams, N. (1984). The psychology of the altruist. *Psychoanalytic Psychology, 1,* 193–213.

McWilliams, N. (1994). *Psychoanalytic diagnosis: Understanding personality structure in the clinical process.* New York: Guilford Press.

McWilliams, N. (1996). Therapy across the sexual orientation boundary: Reflections of a heterosexual female analyst on working with lesbian, gay, and bisexual patients. *Gender and Psychoanalysis, 1,* 203–221.

McWilliams, N. (1998). Relationship, subjectivity, and inference in diagnosis. In J. W. Barron (Ed.), *Making diagnosis meaningful: Enhancing evaluation and treatment of psychological disorders* (pp. 197–226). Washington, DC: American Psychological Association.

Meehl, P. E. (1990). Toward an integrated theory of schizotaxia, schizotypy, and schizophrenia. *Journal of Personality Disorders, 4,* 1–9.

Meissner, W. W. (1978). *The paranoid process.* New York: Aronson.

Meissner, W. W. (1984). *The borderline spectrum: Differential diagnosis and developmental issues.* New York: Aronson.

Meissner, W. W. (1991). *What is effective in psychoanalytic therapy: A move from interpretation to relation.* Northvale, NJ: Aronson.

Meloy, J. R. (1988). *The psychopathic mind: Origins, dynamics, and treatment.* Northvale, NJ: Aronson.

Meloy, J. R. (1992). *Violent attachments.* Northvale, NJ: Aronson.

Meloy, J. R. (1995). Antisocial personality disorder. In G. O. Gabbard (Ed.), *Treatments of psychiatric disorders* (2nd ed., Vol. 2, pp. 2273–2290). Washington, DC: American Psychiatric Press.

Menaker, E. (1953). Masochism—A defense reaction of the ego. *Psychoanalytic Quarterly, 22,* 205–220.

Menaker, E. (1995). *The freedom to inquire: Self psychological perspectives on women's issues, masochism, and the therapeutic relationship.* Northvale, NJ: Aronson.

Messer, S. B. (1994). Adapting psychotherapy outcome research to clinical reality. *Journal of Psychotherapy Integration, 4,* 280–282.

Messer, S. B., & Warren, C. S. (1995). *Models of brief psychodynamic therapy: A comparative approach.* New York: Guilford Press.

Messer, S. B., & Winokur, M. (1980). Some limits to the integration of psychoanalytic and behavior therapy. *American Psychologist, 35,* 818–827.

Messer, S. B., & Wolitzky, D. L. (1997). The traditional psychoanalytic approach to case formulation. In T. D. Eells (Ed.), *Handbook of psychotherapy case formulation* (pp. 26–57). New York: Guilford Press.

Miller, A. (1975). *Prisoners of childhood: The drama of the gifted child and the search for the true self.* New York: Basic Books.

Millon, T. (1981). *Disorders of personality: DSM-III: Axis II.* New York: Wiley.

Mitchell, S. A. (1993). *Hope and dread in psychoanalysis.* New York: Basic Books.

Mitchell, S. A. (1997). *Influence and autonomy in psychoanalysis.* Hillsdale, NJ: Analytic Press.

Mitchell, S. A., & Black, M. J. (1995). *Freud and beyond: A history of modern psychoanalytic thought.* New York: Basic Books.

Modell, A. H. (1975). A narcissistic defense against affects and the illusion of self-sufficiency. *International Journal of Psycho-Analysis, 56,* 275–282.

Money, J. (1988). *Gay, straight, and in-between: The sexology of erotic orientation.* New York: Oxford University Press.

Morgan, A. C. (1997). The application of infant research to psychoanalytic theory and therapy. *Psychoanalytic Psychology, 14,* 315–336.

Morrison, A. P. (1989). *Shame: The underside of narcissism.* Hillsdale, NJ: Analytic Press.

Morrison, J. (1997). *When psychological problems mask medical disorders: A guide for psychotherapists.* New York: Guilford Press.

Moskowitz, M., Monk, C., Kaye, C., & Ellman, S. J. (Eds.). (1997). *The neurobiological and developmental basis for psychotherapeutic intervention.* Northvale, NJ: Aronson.

Mueller, W. J., & Aniskiewitz, A. S. (1986). *Psychotherapeutic intervention in hysterical disorders.* Northvale, NJ: Aronson.

Myers, W. (1984). *Dynamic therapy of the older patient.* New York: Aronson.
Nathan, P. E. (1998). DSM-IV and its antecedents: Enhancing syndromal diagnosis. In J. W. Barron (Ed.), *Making diagnosis meaningful: Enhancing evaluation and treatment of psychological disorders* (pp. 3–27). Washington, DC: American Psychological Association.
Nathanson, D. L. (1990). Project for the study of emotion. In R. A. Glick & S. Bone (Eds.), *Pleasure beyond the pleasure principle: The role of affect in motivation* (pp. 81–110). New Haven, CT: Yale University Press.
Nathanson, D. L. (1992). *Shame and pride: Affect, sex, and the birth of the self.* New York: Norton.
Nemiah, J. C. (1973). *Foundations of psychopathology.* New York: Aronson.
Nemiah, J. C. (1978). Alexithymia and psychosomatic illness. *Journal of Continuing Education in Psychiatry, 25–37.*
Nemiah, J., C., & Sifneos, P. E. (1970). Psychosomatic illness: A problem in communication. *Psychotherapy and Psychosomatics, 18,* 154–160.
Ogden, T. H. (1986). *The matrix of the mind: Object relations and the psychoanalytic dialogue.* Northvale, NJ: Aronson.
Orange, D. M. (1995). *Emotional understanding: Studies in psychoanalytic epistemology.* New York: Guilford Press.
Orange, D. M., Atwood, G. E., & Stolorow, R. D. (1997). *Working intersubjectively: Contextualism in psychoanalytic practice.* Hillsdale, NJ: Analytic Press.
O'Reilly, J. (1972, Spring). The housewife's moment of truth. *Ms.,* pp. 54–59. [Reprinted in *Ms.* (1997, September/October), pp. 16–18.]
Ornstein, P., & Ornstein, A. (1985). Clinical understanding and explaining: The empathic vantage point. In A. Goldberg (Ed.), *Progress in self psychology* (Vol. 1, pp. 43–61). New York: Guilford Press.
Osofsky, J. D. (1995). The effects of exposure to violence on young children. *American Psychologist, 30,* 782–789.
Osofsky, H. J., & Diamond, M. O. (1988). The transition to parenthood: Special tasks and risk factors for adolescent parents. In G. Y. Michaels & W. A. Goldberg (Eds.), *The transition to parenthood: Current theory and research* (pp. 209–234). Cambridge, UK: Cambridge University Press.
Othmer, E., & Othmer, S. C. (1989). *The clinical interview: Using DSM-III-R.* Washington, DC: American Psychiatric Press.
Pally, R. (1998). Emotional processing: The mind–body connection. *International Journal of Psycho-Analysis, 79,* 349–362.
Parkerton, K. (1987). When psychoanalysis is over: An exploration of the psychoanalyst's subjective experience and actual behavior related to the loss of patients at termination and afterward. Unpublished doctoral dissertation, Graduate School of Applied and Professional Psychology, Rutgers University. *Dissertation Abstracts International, 49,* 2790B.
Parloff, M. B. (1982). Psychotherapy research evidence and reimbursement decisions: Bambi meets Godzilla. *American Journal of Psychiatry, 139,* 718–727.
Pennebaker, J. W. (1997). *Opening up: The healing power of expressing emotions.* New York: Guilford Press.
Person, E. S. (1988). *Dreams of love and fateful encounters.* New York: Norton.
Persons, J. B (1991). Psychotherapy outcome studies do not accurately represent current models of psychotherapy. *American Psychologist, 46,* 99–106.
Piaget, J. (1937). *The construction of reality in the child.* New York: Basic Books.

Pine, F. (1985). *Developmental theory and clinical process.* New York: Basic Books.

Pine, F. (1990). *Drive, ego, object, and self: A synthesis for clinical work.* New York: Basic Books.

Pinsker, H. (1997). *A primer of supportive psychotherapy.* Hillsdale, NJ: Analytic Press.

Pope, K. S. (1989). Therapist–patient sex syndrome: A guide for attorneys and subsequent therapists. In G. O. Gabbard (Ed.), *Sexual exploitation in professional relationships* (pp. 39–55). Washington, DC: American Psychiatric Press.

Pruyser, P. W. (1979). *The psychological examination: A guide for clinicians.* New York: International Universities Press.

Putnam, F. W. (1989). *Diagnosis and treatment of multiple personality disorder.* New York: Guilford Press.

Racker, H. (1968). *Transference and countertransference.* New York: International Universities Press.

Rank, O. (1945). *Will therapy and truth and reality.* New York: Knopf.

Rapee, R. M. (1998). *Overcoming shyness and social phobia: A step-by-step guide (clinical application of evidence-based psychotherapy).* Northvale, NJ: Aronson.

Rasmussen, A. (1988). Chronically and severely battered women: A psychodiagnostic investigation. Unpublished doctoral dissertation. Graduate School of Applied and Professional Psychology, Rutgers University. *Dissertation Abstracts International, 50,* 2634B.

Redlich, F. D. (1957). The concept of health in psychiatry. In A. H. Leighton, J. A. Clausen, & R. N. Wilson (Eds.), *Explorations in social psychiatry* (pp. 138–164). New York: Basic Books.

Reich, W. (1933). *Character analysis.* New York: Farrar, Straus, & Giroux, 1972.

Reik, T. (1948). *Listening with the third ear.* New York: Grove.

Richards, H. J. (1993). *Therapy of the substance abuse syndromes.* Northvale, NJ: Aronson.

Robbins, A. (Ed.). (1988). *Between therapists: The processing of transference/countertransference material.* New York: Human Sciences Press.

Robins, L. (1966). *Deviant children grown up: A sociological and psychiatric study of sociopathic personality.* Baltimore: Williams & Wilkins.

Rockland, L. H. (1992a). *Supportive therapy: A psychodynamic approach.* New York: Basic Books.

Rockland, L. H. (1992b). *Supportive therapy for borderline patients: A psychodynamic approach.* New York: Guilford Press.

Rogers, C. R. (1951). *Client-centered therapy: Its current practice, implications, and theory.* Boston: Houghton Mifflin.

Rogers, C. R. (1961). *On becoming a person.* Boston: Houghton Mifflin.

Roland, A. (1981). Induced emotional reactions and attitudes in the psychoanalyst as transference and in actuality. *Psychoanalytic Review, 68,* 45–74.

Roland, A. (1988). *In search of self in India and Japan: Toward a cross-cultural psychology.* Princeton, NJ: Princeton University Press.

Rosenblatt, A. D. (1985). The role of affect in cognitive psychology and psychoanalysis. *Psychoanalytic Psychology, 2,* 85–97.

Rosenthal, D. (1966). *Experimenter effects in behavioral research.* New York: Appleton–Century–Crofts.

Rosenthal, D. (1971). *Genetics of psychopathology*. New York: McGraw-Hill.

Roth, A., & Fonagy, P. (1995, February). *Research on the efficacy and effectiveness of the psychotherapies* (National Health Service Report). London: National Health Services.

Rothstein, A. (1980). *The narcissistic pursuit of perfection*. New York: International Universities Press.

Rowe, C. E., & MacIsaac, D. S. (1989). *Empathic attunement: The "technique" of psychoanalytic self psychology*. Northvale, NJ: Aronson.

Sacks, O. (1990). *Awakenings*. New York: HarperCollins.

Salzman, L. (1980). *Treatment of the obsessive personality*. New York: Aronson.

Sander, L. (1980). New knowledge about the infant from current research: Implications for psychoanalysis. *Journal of the American Psychoanalytic Association, 28*, 181–198.

Sandler, J., & Rosenblatt, B. (1962). The concept of the representational world. *Psychoanalytic Study of the Child, 17*, 128–145.

Sass, L. A. (1992). *Madness and modernism: Insanity in the light of modern art, literature, and thought*. New York: Basic Books.

Saul, L. (1971). *Emotional maturity* (2nd ed.). Philadelphia: Lippincott.

Schafer, R. (1968). *Aspects of internalization*. New York: International Universities Press.

Schafer, R. (1992). *Retelling a life*. New York: Basic Books.

Scharff, D., & Scharff, J. S. (1987). *Object relations family therapy*. Northvale, NJ: Aronson.

Scharff, D., & Scharff, J. S. (1992). *Object relations couple therapy*. Northvale, NJ: Aronson.

Schneider, K. J. (1998). Toward a science of the heart: Romanticism and the revival of psychology. *American Psychologist, 53*, 277–289.

Schofield, W. (1986). *Psychotherapy: The purchase of friendship*. New Brunswick, NJ: Transaction Books.

Schore, A. N. (1994). *Affect regulation and the origin of the self: The neurobiology of emotional development*. New York: Erlbaum.

Schore, A. N. (1997). A century after Freud's Project: Is a rapprochement between psychoanalysis and neurobiology at hand? *Journal of the American Psychoanalytic Association, 45*, 807–840.

Schwartz, R. H. (1991). Heavy marijuana use and recent memory impairment. *Psychiatric Annals, 23*, 80–82.

Searles, H. F. (1959). Oedipal love in the countertransference. In *Collected papers on schizophrenia and other subjects* (pp. 284–303). New York: International Universities Press, 1965.

Sears, R. R., Rau, L., & Alpert, R. (1965). *Identification and child rearing*. Stanford, CA: Stanford University Press.

Seligman, M. (1995). The effectiveness of psychotherapy: The *Consumer Reports* study. *American Psychologist, 50*, 1017–1024.

Seligman, M. (1996). Science as the ally of practice. *American Psychologist, 51*, 1072–1079.

Shane, M., Shane, E., & Gales, M. (1997). *Intimate attachments: Toward a new self psychology*. New York: Guilford Press.

Shapiro, D. (1965). *Neurotic styles*. New York: Basic Books.

Shapiro, F. (1989). *Eye movement desensitization and reprocessing: Basic principles, protocols, and procedures.* New York: Guilford Press.

Share, L. (1994). *If someone speaks, it gets lighter: Dreams and the reconstruction of infant trauma.* Hillsdale, NJ: Analytic Press.

Sifneos, P. E. (1973). The prevalence of "alexithymic" characteristics in psychosomatic patients. *Psychotherapy and Psychosomatics, 22,* 255–262.

Silverman, D. K. (1998). The tie that binds: Affect regulation, attachment, and psychoanalysis. *Psychoanalytic Psychology, 15,* 187–212.

Silverman, L. H. (1984). Beyond insight: An additional necessary step in redressing intrapsychic conflict. *Psychoanalytic Psychology, 1,* 215–234.

Silverman, L. H., Lachmann, F. M., & Milich, R. (1982). *The search for oneness.* New York: International Universities Press.

Singer, E. (1970). *Key concepts in psychotherapy* (2nd ed.). New York: Basic Books.

Slade, A. (1996). Longitudinal studies and clinical psychoanalysis: A view from attachment theory and research. *Journal of Clinical Psychoanalysis, 5,* 112–123.

Smith, M., Glass, G., & Miller, T. (1980). *The benefits of psychotherapy.* Baltimore, MD: Johns Hopkins University Press.

Socarides, D. D., & Stolorow, R. D. (1984–1985). Affects and selfobjects. *Annual of Psychoanalysis, 12/13,* 105–119.

Spence, D. P. (1982). *Narrative truth and historical truth: Meaning and interpretation in psychoanalysis.* New York: Norton.

Spezzano, C. (1993). *Affect in psychoanalysis: A clinical synthesis.* Hillsdale, NJ: Analytic Press.

Spiegel, D., Bloom, J., Kraemer, H., & Gottheil, E. (1989). Effects of psychosocial treatment on survival of patients with metastatic breast cancer. *The Lancet, ii* (8668), 888–891.

Spitz, R. (1945). Hospitalism. An inquiry into the genesis of psychiatric conditions in early childhood. *Psychoanalytic Study of the Child, 1,* 53–74.

Stark, M. (1994). *Working with resistance.* Northvale, NJ. Aronson.

Stern, D. B. (1997). *Unformulated experience: From dissociation to imagination in psychoanalysis.* Hillsdale, NJ: Analytic Press.

Stern, D. N. (1985). *The interpersonal world of the infant: A view from psychoanalysis and developmental psychology.* New York: Basic Books.

Stern, D. N. (1995). *The motherhood constellation: A unified view of parent–infant psychotherapy.* New York: Basic Books.

Stolorow, R. D. (1975). The narcissistic function of masochism (and sadism). *International Journal of Psycho-Analysis, 56,* 441–448.

Stolorow, R. D., & Atwood, G. E. (1979). *Faces in a cloud. Subjectivity in personality theory.* New York: Aronson. (Rev. ed. 1993.)

Stolorow, R. D., & Atwood, G. E. (1992). *Contexts of being: The intersubjective foundations of psychological life.* Hillsdale, NJ: Analytic Press.

Stolorow, R. D., Brandshaft, B. & Atwood, G. E. (1987). *Psychoanalytic treatment: An intersubjective approach.* Hillsdale, NJ: Analytic Press.

Stolorow, R. D., & Lachmann, F. M.(1980). *Psychoanalysis of developmental arrests: Theory and treatment.* New York: International Universities Press.

Stosney, S. (1995). *Treating attachment abuse: A compassionate approach.* New York: Springer.

Strachey, J. (1934). The nature of the therapeutic action of psycho-analysis. *International Journal of Psycho-Analysis, 15,* 127–159.

Stricker, G. (1996, October 24). Untitled address to faculty and students at the Graduate School of Applied and Professional Psychology, Rutgers University, Piscataway, NJ.

Strupp, H. H. (1996). The tripartite model and the *Consumer Reports* study. *American Psychologist, 51,* 1017–1024.

Sue, D. W., & Sue, D. (1990). *Counseling the culturally different: Theory and practice* (2nd ed.). New York: Wiley.

Sulloway, F. J. (1979). *Freud, biologist of the mind: Beyond the psychoanalytic legend.* New York: Basic Books.

Sullivan, H. S. (1947). *Conceptions of modern psychiatry.* New York: Norton.

Sullivan, H. S. (1953). *Interpersonal theory of psychiatry.* New York: Norton.

Sullivan, H. S. (1954). *The psychiatric interview.* New York: Norton.

Terr, L. (1992). *Too scared to cry: Psychic trauma in childhood.* New York: HarperCollins.

Terr, L. (1993). *Unchained memories: True stories of traumatic memories, lost and found.* New York: Basic Books.

Thomas, A., Chess, S., & Birch, H. G. (1968). *Temperament and behavior disorders in children.* New York: New York University Press.

Thompson, C. L. (1996). The African-American patient in psychodynamic treatment. In R. P. Foster, M. Moskowitz, & R. A. Javier (Eds.), *Reaching across boundaries of culture and class: Widening the scope of psychotherapy* (pp. 115–142). Northvale, NJ: Aronson.

Tomkins, S. S. (1962). *Affect, imagery, consciousness: Vol. 1. The positive affects.* New York: Springer.

Tomkins, S. S. (1963). *Affect, imagery, consciousness: Vol. 2. The negative affects.* New York: Springer.

Tomkins, S. S. (1982). Affect theory. In P. Ekman (Ed.), *Emotion in the human face* (2nd ed., pp. 353–395). New York: Cambridge University Press.

Tomkins, S. S. (1991). *Affect, imagery, consciousness: Vol. 3. The negative affects: Anger and fear.* New York: Springer.

Trevarthen, C. (1980). The foundations of intersubjectivity: Development of interpersonal and cooperative understanding in infants. In D. R. Olsen (Ed.), *The social foundation of language and thought: Essays in honor of Jerome Bruner* (pp. 316–342). New York: Norton.

Trevino, F., & Rendon, M. (1994). Mental health of Latinos in the United States. In C. Molina & M. Molina-Aguirre (Eds.), *Latino health in the United States: A growing challenge* (pp. 447–475). Washington, DC: American Public Health Association.

Tronick, E., Als, H., & Brazelton, T. B. (1977). The infant's capacity to regulate mutuality in face-to-face interaction. *Journal of Communication, 27,* 74–80.

Trop, J. L. (1988). Erotic and eroticized transference—A self psychology perspective. *Psychoanalytic Psychology, 5,* 269–284.

Tyson, P., & Tyson, R. L. (1990). *Psychoanalytic theories of development: An integration.* New Haven, CT: Yale University Press.

Vaillant, G. E. (1971). Theoretical hierarchy of adaptive ego mechanisms. *Archives of General Psychiatry, 24,* 107–118.

Vaillant, G. E. (1977). *Adaptation to life.* Boston: Little, Brown.

Vaillant, G. E. (1992). *Ego mechanisms of defense.* Washington, DC: American Psychiatric Press.

Vaillant, G. E., & McCullough, L. (1998). The role of ego mechanisms of defense in the diagnosis of personality disorders. In J. W. Barron (Ed.), *Making diagnosis meaningful: Enhancing evaluation and treatment of psychological disorders* (pp. 139–158). Washington, DC: American Psychological Association.

VandenBos, G. R., (Ed.). (1986). Psychotherapy research: A special issue. *American Psychologist, 41,* 111–112.

VandenBos, G. R. (Ed.). (1996). Outcome assessment of psychotherapy [Special issue]. *American Psychologist, 51.*

van der Kolk, B. A. (1994). The body keeps the score: Memory and the evolving psychobiology of posttraumatic stress. *Harvard Review of Psychiatry, 1,* 253–265.

Vaughan, S. C. (1997). *The talking cure: The science behind psychotherapy.* New York: Putnam.

Viorst, J. (1986). *Necessary losses: The loves, illusions, dependencies and impossible expectations that all of us have to give up in order to grow.* New York: Simon & Schuster.

Wachtel, P. L. (1977). *Psychoanalysis and behavior therapy: Toward an integration.* New York: Basic Books.

Wachtel, P. L., & Messer, S. B. (1997). *Theories of psychotherapy: Origins and evolution.* Washington, DC: American Psychological Association.

Waelder, R. (1960). *Basic theory of psychoanalysis.* New York: International Universities Press.

Wallerstein, J. S., & Blakeslee, S. (1989). *Second chances: Men, women, and children a decade after divorce.* New York: Ticknor & Fields.

Wallerstein, R. S. (1986). *Forty-two lives in treatment: A study of psychoanalysis and psychotherapy.* New York: Guilford Press.

Watson, J. B. (1925). *Behaviorism.* New York: People's Institute Publishing Co.

Weinstock, A. (1967). A longitudinal study of social class and defense. *Journal of Consulting Psychology, 31,* 539–541.

Weiss, J. (1993). *How psychotherapy works: Process and technique.* New York: Guilford Press.

Weiss, J., Sampson, H., & the Mount Zion Psychotherapy Research Group. (1986). *The psychoanalytic process: Theory, clinical observations, and empirical research.* New York: Guilford Press.

Welch, B. L. (1998, August 15). *The assault on managed care: Why long-term intensive treatment will survive.* Paper presented at the 106th annual meeting of the American Psychological Association, San Francisco, CA.

Westen, D. (1998). Case formulation and personality diagnosis: Two processes or one? In J. W. Barron (Ed.), *Making diagnosis meaningful: Enhancing evaluation and treatment of psychological disorders* (pp. 111–137). Washington, DC: American Psychological Association.

Whitson, G. (1996). Working-class issues. In R. P. Foster, M. Moskowitz, & R. A. Javier (Eds.), *Reaching across boundaries of culture and class: Widening the scope of psychotherapy* (pp. 143–157). Northvale, NJ: Aronson.

Wilson, A. (1995). Mapping the mind in relational psychoanalysis: Some critiques, questions, and conjectures. *Psychoanalytic Psychology, 12,* 9–30.

Wilson, A., & Prillaman, J. (1997). Early development and disorders of internalization. In Moskowitz, M., Monk, C., Kaye, C., & Ellman, S. J. (Eds.), *The neurobiological basis for psychotherapeutic intervention* (pp. 189–233). Northvale, NJ: Aronson.

Winnicott, D. W. (1965). *The maturational process and the facilitating environment.* New York: International Universities Press.

Wolf, E. (1988). *Treating the self: Elements of clinical self psychology.* New York: Guilford Press.

Wolff, P. H. (1970). *The developmental psychologies of Jean Piaget and psychoanalysis.* New York: International Universities Press.

Wolff, P. H. (1996). The irrelevance of infant observation for psychoanalysis. *Journal of the American Psychoanalytic Association, 44,* 369–392.

Zeanah, C., Anders, T., Seifer, R., & Stern, D. N. (1989). Implications of research on infant development for psychodynamic theory and practice. *Journal of the American Academy of Child and Adolescent Development, 28,* 657–668.

Zimbardo, P. G. (1990). *Shyness: What it is, what to do about it.* New York: Perseus Press.

Zubin, J., & Spring, B. (1977). Vulnerability—a new view of schizophrenia. *Journal of Abnormal Psychology, 86,* 103–126.

Author Index

Subject Index